GOVERNORS STATE UNIVERSITY LIBRARY

MW00386670

Governors State University
Library Hours
Monday thru Thursday 8:00 to 10:30
Friday 8:00 to 5:00
Saturday 8:30 to 5:00
Sunday 1:00 to 5:00 (Fall
and Winter Trimester Only)

WITHDRAWN

The Dilemma of Federal
Mental Health Policy

GOVERNORS STATE UNIVERSITY
UNIVERSITY PARK
IL 60466

Critical Issues in Health and Medicine

Edited by Rima D. Apple, University of Wisconsin–Madison, and Janet Golden, Rutgers University, Camden

Growing criticism of the U.S. healthcare system is coming from consumers, politicians, the media, activists, and healthcare professionals. Critical Issues in Health and Medicine is a collection of books that explores these contemporary dilemmas from a variety of perspectives, among them political, legal, historical, sociological, and comparative, and with attention to crucial dimensions such as race, gender, ethnicity, sexuality, and culture.

The Dilemma of Federal Mental Health Policy

Radical Reform or Incremental Change?

Gerald N. Grob and Howard H. Goldman

GOVERNORS STATE UNIVERSITY
UNIVERSITY PARK
IL 60466

Rutgers University Press

New Brunswick, New Jersey, and London

RA
790.6
.G76
2006

Library of Congress Cataloging-in-Publication Data

Grob, Gerald N., 1931–

The dilemma of federal mental health policy : radical reform or incremental change? / Gerald N. Grob and Howard H. Goldman.

p. ; cm. — (Critical issues in health and medicine)

Includes bibliographical references and index.

ISBN-13: 978-0-8135-3958-4 (hardcover : alk. paper)

ISBN-10: 0-8135-3958-7 (hardcover : alk. paper)

1. Federal aid to community mental health services.   2. Mental health services.
3. Health care reform.   4. Medical policy.   I. Goldman, Howard H.   II. Title.   III. Series.

[DNLM: 1. Mental Health Services—United States.   2. Health Care Reform—United States.   3. Health Policy—United States.   4. Legislation, Medical—United States.   WM 30 G873d 2006]

RA790.6.G76   2006

362.1'0425—dc22   2006919751

A British Cataloging-in-Publication record for this book is available from the British Library

Copyright © 2006 by Gerald N. Grob and Howard H. Goldman

All rights reserved

No part of this book may be reproduced or utilized in any form or by any means, electronic or mechanical, or by any information storage and retrieval system, without written permission from the publisher. Please contact Rutgers University Press, 100 Joyce Kilmer Avenue, Piscataway, NJ 08854–8099. The only exception to this prohibition is "fair use" as defined by U.S. copyright law.

Manufactured in the United States of America

Contents

Preface

This book is a collaborative work by a historian (Gerald N. Grob) and a psychiatrist (Howard H. Goldman). At first glance our respective disciplines appear to be far apart. Appearances, however, can be deceiving. Both of us have spent much of our careers studying mental health policy, the role of government (local, state, and national), the practice of psychiatry and allied mental health disciplines, and, above all, the fate of individuals with severe and persistent mental illnesses. We have been fascinated by the claims of successive generations that their policies would resolve the pressing needs of individuals whose severe mental illnesses have often created dependency and thus required either public or private assistance. What is equally fascinating is the fact that many "solutions" have embodied an ideological agenda that often lacked any basis in reality and ignored available empirical data.

This book attempts to trace the evolution of *federal* mental health policy from World War II to the beginning of the twenty-first century. These decades have been marked by a determined effort both to shift the locus of policy away from institutional to community care and to transfer leadership and authority from the states to the federal government. As a result of America's peculiar federal system, intergovernmental rivalries and efforts to shift costs to different levels of government have played an important if overlooked part in the transfer of power and the reshaping of policy. In recent decades, moreover, policy outcomes have often reflected the actions of federal bureaucrats who are responsible for developing the guidelines to implement legislation. At the same time the growing preoccupation with psychological maladjustment and the creation of myriad diagnostic categories have also brought new groups into the mental health arena. The decline of traditional mental hospital care and the rise of a community care policy, paradoxically, created a fragmented rather than a unified mental health system. Those most in need–persons with severe disorders–have often proved to be the losers.

In tracing the history of mental health policy, we have emphasized intergovernmental relationships and the rise of federal authority. We could have written a separate volume about *state* mental health policy, since that is where many of the innovations in services and government stewardship of mental health have occurred during the same time period. But we have focused on federal policy, if only because many state and local innovations have come in response to changing federal rules and regulations and the incentives associated with them. We also address a theme that resonates in the making of not only mental health policy but other policies as well, namely, what kinds of tactics and strategies tend to have the most concrete and beneficial results? Advocates of radical reform have insisted upon the necessity of fundamental changes. Their efforts were crowned with the passage of the Community Mental Health Acts of 1963 and 1965. These two pieces of federal legislation had two basic objectives: first, to replace archaic and obsolete mental hospitals that had presumably outlived their usefulness; second, to create a radically new institution—the community mental health center—that would benefit individuals with severe and persistent mental disorders. By contrast, other advocates emphasized the importance of smaller incremental changes. They were instrumental in the formulation of the National Plan for the Chronically Mentally Ill in late 1980, a plan that employed resources from a number of federal entitlement laws as well as Medicaid and Medicare to alleviate the problems faced by individuals with severe disorders. The debates over tactics and strategy and the policy consequences that followed illuminate not merely mental health policy but general health policy as well.

Portions of chapters 3 and 4 are reprinted, in revised form, from Gerald N. Grob, "Public Policy and Mental Illnesses: Jimmy Carter's Presidential Commission on Mental Health," *Milbank Quarterly* 83, no. 3 (2005): 425–456.

In writing this book we have drawn on the work of many scholars whose contributions are listed in the notes. We would also like to thank Bernard Arons, Richard Frank, Dolly Gattozzi, Sherry Glied, Michael Hogan, Chris Koyanagi, David Mechanic, Joseph Morrissey, Leonard Rubenstein, and Steven S. Sharfstein, who have reviewed drafts or collaborated on important documents that served as the basis for much of our analysis. HHG would like to acknowledge support from the John D. and Catherine T. MacArthur Foundation Network on Mental Health Policy Research. We also want to recognize the contributions of Carl A. Taube, whose untimely death in 1989 meant that he would not live to see the impact of his creativity in stimulating the developing field of mental health services research and economics.

Gerald N. Grob
Howard H. Goldman

Abbreviations

ACCESS   Access to Community Care and Effective Services and Supports

ACT   Assertive Community Treatment

ADAMHA   Alcohol, Drug Abuse, and Mental Health Administration

AFDC   Aid to Families with Dependent Children

AFSCME   American Federation of State, County, and Municipal Employees

AHCPR   Agency for Health Care Policy and Research

AHRQ   Agency for Healthcare Research and Quality

AMA   American Medical Association

APA   American Psychiatric Association

CHAMPUS   Civilian Health and Medical Program of the Uniformed Services

CMHC   Community Mental Health Center

COBRA   Comprehensive Omnibus Budget Reconciliation Act

CSP   Community Support Program

DHEW   Department of Health, Education, and Welfare

DHHS   Department of Health and Human Services

DRG   Diagnosis-Related Group

EPSDT   Early Periodic Screening, Diagnosis, and Treatment

ERISA   Employee Retirement Income Security Act of 1974

FEHB   Federal Employees Health Benefit Program

GAO   General Accounting Office (later General Accountability Office)

HCFA   Health Care Financing Administration

HUD   Department of Housing and Urban Development

ICD   International Classification of Diseases

JCMIH	Joint Commission on Mental Illness and Health
NAMI	National Alliance for the Mentally Ill
NIAAA	National Institute on Alcohol Abuse and Alcoholism
NIDA	National Institute on Drug Abuse
NIH	National Institutes of Health
NIMH	National Institute of Mental Health
OBRA	Omnibus Budget Reconciliation Act
OMB	Office of Management and Budget
PCMH	President's Commission on Mental Health
PHS	Public Health Service
PPS	Prospective Payment System
RWJF	Robert Wood Johnson Foundation
SAMHSA	Substance Abuse and Mental Health Services Administration
SSA	Social Security Administration
SSDI	Social Security Disability Insurance
SSI	Supplementary Security Income for the Aged, the Disabled, and the Blind

The Dilemma of Federal
Mental Health Policy

Prologue

Lunacy, insanity, mental illnesses—whatever the term or diagnostic category—have seemingly been an omnipresent feature of the human condition. Virtually every society has been forced to confront the presence of persons whose aberrant behavior and condition invariably led to dependency. For families such members created a variety of tragic problems that were often intractable in nature. Community reaction was equally problematic, and ranged from fear, stigmatization, and a desire to exclude, on the one hand, to sympathy, on the other.

That such persons were generally unable to survive on their own raised grave problems. What was the responsibility of the family? Could families be required to provide care when the presence of such persons in a household threatened to destroy its integrity? Did the community have a moral obligation to ensure the safety and well-being of such persons if the family was unable to do so, assuming even that the person had a family? If so, what kinds of arrangements could ensure that such individuals would be provided with the basic necessities of life that were required for survival? What groups were most qualified to provide authoritative solutions? What level of government should assume primary responsibility?

Such questions have been answered in very different ways. Sometimes neglect has been characteristic; sometimes communities have developed ad hoc mechanisms to ensure minimal access to the basic necessities of life; and at other times confinement in institutions such as almshouses, jails, and hospitals has been common. What is striking is the absence of any consensus on the underlying causes responsible for the behaviors that have provoked these reactions. Causation has been attributed to individual misbehavior, to broad social, economic, and environmental factors, to underlying focal infections or physiological disorders, and to chemical imbalances, to cite only a few explanations. Nor has the medicalization of insanity resolved differences; the disagreements among psychiatrists (to say nothing about other mental health professionals) are as pronounced as those among the general public.

Serious and persistent mental disorders remain among the most pressing health and social problems in contemporary America. Recent estimates suggest that the total number of persons with these disorders may run as high as 3 million; the direct and indirect costs of their care and treatment run into the tens of billions of dollars. The human and social dimensions of the problem are staggering. Persons with serious disorders find that their ability to cope with daily life is severely impaired and that economic self-sufficiency becomes virtually impossible. Their inescapable presence poses tragic choices for themselves, their families, and society generally.

For nearly two centuries Americans have grappled with the dilemmas posed by the presence of persons with severe psychiatric disorders. In the nineteenth century states created an extensive public mental hospital system and allocated significant funds for its support. During the second half of the twentieth century a reaction against institutional care was accompanied by claims both that community care and treatment represented a superior policy choice and that the federal government—not the states—should shape policy. Yet at the beginning of the twenty-first century the plight of many persons with severe and persistent mental disorders remains as pressing as ever.

That the federal government would play a major role in mental health could not have been predicted. Before 1800 mental illnesses were neither defined in medical terms nor identified as a pressing social problem. A predominantly rural society cared for "distracted" persons or "lunaticks"—to employ seventeenth- and eighteenth-century terminology—in a variety of informal ways and within the framework of either existing poor laws, private charity, or a combination of both. There is little evidence, moreover, to substantiate the oft-repeated allegation that persons with severe mental disorders were singled out for unduly harsh and inhumane treatment. Given prevailing standards of living, available resources, and the absence of formal institutions, there is no reason to suggest that the fate of the insane was appreciably different from other groups whose condition created dependency. Fiscal concerns, though omnipresent, were modified by long-standing ethical and moral values that were predicated on the assumption that society had an obligation to assist those unable to survive independently.[1]

In the early nineteenth century, however, a profound transformation occurred in the ways Americans perceived mental illnesses and in the priorities they set for the care of afflicted persons. In brief, the older and ad hoc ways in which local communities had dealt with mental disorders were partially abandoned and were replaced by a policy that emphasized a novel institution—the asylum, retreat, or mental hospital. Nowhere was the enthusiasm for institutional care better stated than in Dorothea L. Dix's impassioned memorials pleading with states legislatures to create public mental hospitals. "I come to present the strong claims of suffering humanity," she informed the members of the Massachusetts legislature in her first memorial in 1843. "I come as the advocate of helpless, forgotten, insane and idiotic men and women; of beings, sunk to a condition from which the most unconcerned would start with real horror." In New Jersey Dix found "in jails and poorhouses, and wandering at will over the country, large numbers of insane and idiotic persons." Such a state of affairs, she told the Tennessee legislature four years later, was inexcusable, since the remedy was available in the form of "*rightly organized Hospitals*, adapted to the special care of the peculiar malady of the Insane."[2]

The creation of institutions reflected an extraordinarily optimistic view of the nature and prognosis of mental illnesses. Since insanity was thought to follow improper behavioral patterns associated with a defective environment, therapy had to begin with the creation of a new and presumably more appropriate environment. Hospitalization was a sine qua non because it shattered the link between an improper environment and the patient. In a hospital patients could be exposed to a judicious amalgam of medical and moral treatment. The former was designed to rebuild the body to improve the mind and to calm violent behavior by the administration of narcotics. "Moral treatment"—to use nineteenth-century terminology—implied kind, individualized care within a small hospital. It involved occupational therapy, religious exercises, amusements, and games. There were to be no threats of physical violence, and only rarely were mechanical means of restraint to be employed. Moral treatment, in effect, involved the re-education of the patient within a more appropriate environment and assumed that mental disorders were, in the early stages, curable. Conversely, chronicity was neither inherent nor inevitable, but followed the failure to provide acute cases with the benefits of therapy in hospitals.

In the decades following the appearance of such institutions in the 1820s and 1830s virtually every state established one or more public mental hospitals, which were widely regarded as the symbol of an enlightened and progressive nation that no longer ignored or mistreated its insane citizens. The justification for these hospitals appeared self-evident: they benefited the community, the family, and the individual by offering effective medical treatment for acute cases and humane custodial care for chronic cases. In providing for persons with mental illnesses, states met an ethical and moral responsibility and, at the same time, contributed to the general welfare by limiting, if not eliminating, the spread of disease and dependency. The founding of mental hospitals was but one indication of a shift in authority away from local communities and toward greater intervention by states. Indeed, the social, economic, and technological changes that were beginning to transform American society in the antebellum decades were accompanied by a rapid expansion in the activities of most state governments, which took an active, if not dominant, role in formulating welfare policies and regulating economic development.

For more than a century the care and treatment of persons with mental illnesses remained overwhelmingly a state responsibility. In part this state of affairs grew out of America's federal structure. The writing and ratification of the Constitution reflected colonial anger at the centralized and seemingly arbitrary rule by the British government. The founding fathers, therefore, decided to restrict the functions of the new national government and to reserve a large reservoir of power for the states. The tenth amendment explicitly stated that the "powers not delegated to the United States by the Constitution . . . [are] reserved to the States, respectively, or to the people." However the document is interpreted, it is clear that its authors believed that responsibility for health and welfare resided with local and state governments, not with the federal government. An early effort to use federal largesse came to naught. In 1854 a presidential veto of a congressional act setting aside 10 million acres to be used by states for indigent persons with mental disorders ensured that the national government would not intrude in health and welfare policy. The first major intrusion of the federal government into the welfare arena came with the enactment of a program to assist veterans of the Civil War. By the turn of the century it had been transformed into a universal disability and old age program for veterans and their dependents. About 25 percent of all those aged sixty-five and over were enrolled. By 1885 the costs of this program accounted for just over a quarter of all federal expenditures and, a decade later, reached a high of over 40 percent.[3]

Responsibility for the care of persons with mental disorders by states meant that the policymaking process was decentralized and that variability was characteristic. New York and Massachusetts, for example, had geographically dispersed hospitals and the highest per capita expenditures in the nineteenth century and the early part of the twentieth. The lowest per capita expenditures, by contrast, were in the South. This pattern persisted for over a century. In 1940 the average per capita expenditure for the nation as a whole was $301. The comparable averages for New England, the Mid-Atlantic, the South Atlantic, and the East South Central were $388, $377, $269, and $172, respectively.[4] Lower expenditures in the South were in part a function of the region's widespread poverty. But slavery and the pattern of segregation that emerged by the end of the nineteenth century created a political structure that tended to minimize social welfare expenditures. The quality and quantity of care, noted Joseph Zubin and Grace C. Scholz in their 1940 analysis of regional differences, was directly related to per capita expenditures.[5] A decentralized political structure resulted in wide disparities in the policies and practices of different states. As long as mental health policy was the responsibility of states, formidable barriers would complicate efforts to introduce fundamental changes.

The founding of state mental hospitals did not occur in a social or political vacuum. The tradition of local autonomy that had grown out of nearly two centuries of colonial experience continued to influence both the creation and the administration of welfare policies. Many of the early state laws pertaining to insanity, therefore, were based on the assumption that policy had to embody shared responsibilities with local communities. Thus the older tradition of local autonomy continued to play an important policy role, even at a time when rapid social and economic change pointed toward greater centralization.

State legislatures generally provided the capital funds necessary for acquiring a hospital site, constructing the physical plant, and often even paying the salaries of superintendents and other officers. Local communities, by contrast, were required to reimburse the hospital for the cost of caring for and treating their residents. The system, moreover, did not assume that all persons with a mental disorder would be cared for in state institutions. A high priority was set on committing persons whose disorder rendered them dangerous to themselves or others. Those who could presumably benefit from a therapeutic regimen could be committed at the discretion of local officials. Indeed, no matter how large the institutionalized population, more persons with mental disorders remained in the community, residing either at home or in an almshouse. In short, the system involved dual responsibility, even though states assumed the costs of patients who lacked a legal residence (for example, immigrants).

The division of responsibility between local and state governments for persons with mental disorders had significant repercussions. Intergovernmental rivalries played major roles in shaping policy both in the nineteenth century and in the second half of the twentieth century, when the federal government began to play an increasingly dominant role. A political system with divided responsibility tended to promote competition and rivalries that were inherent in overlapping jurisdictions. The stipulation that communities were financially liable for the support of residents with mental illnesses created an incentive to retain them in local almshouses, where per capita costs were much lower. If states assumed greater fiscal responsibilities for such persons, localities were more prone to commit residents to state facilities. Funding patterns in many states played a decisive role in determining whether persons who were mentally disordered would be placed in asylums, almshouses, or simply left on their own.

Nor were state hospitals unaffected by the prevailing division of authority. Patient fees, generally set by legislatures, were often insufficient or marginal; slow and delinquent payments by local officials resulted in cash-flow problems; and inadequate or tardy state appropriations further compounded individual institutional problems. Hospital officials sometimes faced unremitting local pressure to discharge their residents irrespective of therapeutic considerations. In a few extreme cases, local officials inaugurated legal proceedings against hospital authorities in the hope of recouping money for the labor of their patients even though such work was part of a therapeutic regimen.[6]

Aware of the problems arising out of divided authority, some states—particularly those in the more recently settled western areas—assumed responsibility for all the costs of hospital care. By 1860 Ohio, Indiana, Illinois, Wisconsin, and California paid the full costs of hospitalization; six other states, in contrast, limited their support only to indigent patients.[7] Others adopted variations, including an annual fixed appropriation. Although such modifications eased tensions, they failed to resolve existing difficulties, if only because there were always more patients than hospital beds. This situation led local communities to develop their own ways of providing care for their dependent residents with mental disorders.

Beneath the rhetoric that accompanied debates over the proper configuration of public policy lay a series of complex issues. Did the steady increase in hospital populations undermine therapeutic goals? Given rising pressures to admit new individuals with disorders as well as the expectation that hospitals would allow patients who did not improve or recover to accumulate, should additional facilities be built? Should local communities continue to retain responsibility for persons with mental disorders who were placed in almshouses or other welfare institutions? What level of government—local or state—should bear the greatest burden of support?

The answers varied widely. In 1869 New York, for example, opened the Willard Hospital for the Chronic Insane, which was intended to care for all chronic patients. But Willard was not equal to the task. Within a few years the legislature enacted the Exempted Counties Act to permit localities to maintain their own institutions. Wisconsin set up a system of county asylums for long-stay patients and provided a partial subsidy for their care, thus in theory permitting state hospitals to focus on therapy. Eclectic approaches were characteristic. Friction between local and state officials over the allocation of fiscal responsibilities was also characteristic, but funding was by no means the only source of conflict. On the one hand, local officials responsible for the care of dependent groups argued that persons with persistent mental illnesses ought not to be sent to geographically distant state hospitals where they were isolated from family and other personal ties. State officials and other professional and organizationally minded individuals, on the other hand, believed that preoccupation with costs ensured that local care would always remain substandard.[8]

Toward the close of the nineteenth century, coalitions that included physicians and social welfare activists began to lobby for an end to dual responsibility. New York led the way in 1890 with the passage of its influential State Care Act, which mandated that persons with mental illnesses were to be wards of the state. Over time virtually all states followed suit, thus absolving most localities of any responsibility. Those who favored centralization believed that local care, though less expensive, was not only substandard but also fostered chronicity and dependency. Conversely, care and treatment in hospitals, though initially more costly, was thought to be cheaper in the long run because it would enhance the odds of recovery for some and provide more humane care for others.[9]

The assumption by states of responsibility for persons with mental illnesses, however, had completely unpredictable consequences that presaged a shift in the character of hospital populations. Between the 1830s and the 1880s, the proportion of long-term or chronic cases in hospitals was relatively low in comparison with the extraordinary high percentage between 1890 and 1950. Funding patterns had played a key role in hastening change. In brief, local officials saw in the new laws a golden opportunity to shift some of their financial obligations onto state governments. The purpose of the legislation mandating a state takeover was self-evident, namely, to remove the care of persons with persistent mental illnesses from local jurisdictions. But local officials went well beyond the intent of the law. Traditionally, nineteenth-century almshouses (which were supported and administered by local governments) served in part as old-age homes for senile and aged persons without any financial resources. The passage of state care acts provided local officials with an unexpected opportunity. They redefined senility in psychiatric terms and thus began to send aged persons to state mental hospitals rather than to almshouses. Humanitarian concerns played a relatively minor role in this development; economic considerations were paramount.[10] Between 1880 and 1920, therefore, the almshouse populations (for this and other reasons) dropped precipitously. What occurred, however, was not a deinstitutionalization movement but rather a lateral transfer of individuals between institutions.

The successful effort by local communities to shift costs to the states was not unique. The American political system, for better or worse, maximizes attempts to devolve costs to higher as well as to lower levels of government. In the late nineteenth century and the early twentieth local governments made determined efforts to have state governments assume some of their functions. After World War II, states were more than happy to take advantage of federal programs and subsidies in the hope of reducing their own outlays. In the late twentieth century the pattern began to be reversed, as the federal government began to devolve some of its responsibilities downward to the states and local communities. From an economic point of view, such cost shifting made little sense; from a political point of view it was understandable.

During the first half of the twentieth century the character of mental hospitals underwent a dramatic transformation as a result of changes in governmental responsibilities. By 1904, only 28 percent of the total patient population had been institutionalized for twelve months or less. Six years later this percentage fell to 13, although it rose to 17 in 1923. The greatest change came among patients hospitalized for five years or more. In 1904, 39 percent of patients fell into this category; in 1910 and 1923 the respective percentages were 52 and 54.[11] Although data for the United States as a whole are unavailable after 1923, the experiences of Massachusetts are illustrative. By the 1930s nearly 80 percent of the state's mental hospital beds were occupied by patients with chronic mental disorders.[12] Chronicity, however, is a somewhat misleading term, for the group that it described was actually heterogeneous. The aged (over sixty or sixty-five) constituted by far the single largest component. As late as 1958 nearly a third of all resident state mental hospital patients were over sixty-five.[13]

The increase in long-stay patients—which resulted from the redefinition of senility in psychiatric terms—tended to reinforce the perception that hospitals were merely serving a custodial role. This perception was strengthened by the Great Depression of the 1930s and World War II; both led to a fall in the quality of institutional care because of the decline in state appropriations in the 1930s and the loss of professional personnel during the war. Yet appearances were somewhat deceiving, for a substantial number of patients were discharged after relatively short hospital stays. In a study of more than 15,000 patients admitted for the first time to Warren State Hospital in Pennsylvania during the period from 1916 to 1950, Morton Kramer and his associates found marked improvements in the release rates of the cohorts of 1936–1945 and 1946–1950, as compared with those of 1916–1925 and 1926–1935. A comparison of the earliest and latest cohorts indicated that the probability of being released within a year of admission increased from 42 to 62 percent. Subsequent studies revealed that the experiences of Warren State Hospital were by no means atypical, a finding suggesting that some patients continued to benefit from hospitalization. Although release from the hospital was not synonymous with recovery, it meant that the individual could reside in the community.[14]

At the same time that the nature of the mental hospital resident population was changing, American psychiatry was undergoing a fundamental transformation. Between 1890 and 1940 psychiatrists began to look beyond the institutions in which their specialty had been conceived. Nineteenth-century psychiatrists had emphasized managerial and administrative issues, and in so doing had made the care of institutionalized patients their primary responsibility. Their twentieth-century successors, by contrast, looked beyond the institutions that had for so long defined their specialty. The rise of modern "scientific" medicine only strengthened their desire to create a new kind of psychiatry. Under such circumstances, it was understandable that psychiatrists between 1890 and World War II began to redefine not only concepts of mental disorders and therapeutic interventions but the very context in which they practiced. In so doing, they began to distance themselves from traditional mental hospitals which—unlike their nineteenth-century predecessors—had large numbers of chronic and aged patients whose need for general care was paramount. The effort to shift the foundations of psychiatric practice seemed appropriate in view of the widespread, if inaccurate, belief that scientific medicine was responsible for the decline in mortality from infectious diseases and the increase in life expectancy at birth. By identifying with general medicine, psychiatrists slowly began to shift the location of their practice from mental hospitals to outpatient facilities, child guidance clinics, private practice, and general hospitals. After 1945 this trend would be vastly accelerated. The creation of new federal programs would also alter the very foundations of psychiatric and mental health practice.[15]

Another visible symbol of change was the creation of a mental hygiene movement after 1900. Reflecting a commitment to science, mental hygienists saw disease as a product of environmental, hereditary, and individual deficiencies; its eradication required a fusion of scientific and administrative action. As members of a profession they believed was destined to play an increasingly central role in the creation of a new social order, psychiatrists began to redefine their role. The emphasis on scientific research rather than on care or custody, on disease rather than patients, and on alternatives to the traditional mental hospital was merely a beginning. More compelling was the utopian idea of a society structured in a way that would maximize health and minimize disease. The founding of the National Committee for Mental Hygiene in 1909 was a visible symbol of change. The new psychiatry, insisted Dr. Thomas W. Salmon (the committee's first medical director), had to reach beyond institutional walls and play a crucial part "in the great movements for social betterment." Psychiatrists could no longer limit their activities and responsibilities to the institutionalized mentally ill. On the contrary, they had to lead the way in research and policy formulation and to develop mechanisms to promote mental hygiene goals. Their responsibilities, he added, included the care of the feebleminded, the control of alcoholism, the management of abnormal children, the treatment of criminals, the fostering of eugenics, and the prevention of crime, prostitution, and dependency.[16]

The effort to define alternative career roles, however, did not create a specialty where consensus rather than conflict was characteristic of practice and theory. Some psychiatrists emphasized brain pathology; others insisted that focal infections in any part of the body could lead to mental illnesses; others centered their attention on the role of the endocrine system; and still others emphasized the importance of understanding the manner in which the individual's life history shaped maladaptive traits that gave rise to mental disorders.

Therapies were equally eclectic. By the 1930s insulin and electric shock therapy, psychosurgery, and a variety of psychotherapies existed side by side. The
absence of theoretical rationales for many therapies was not unrecognized. "At
present," noted the authors of a leading text, "we can only say that we are treating empirically disorders whose etiology is unknown with shock treatments
whose action is also shrouded in mystery."[17]

The creation of both a new kind of psychiatry and a mental hygiene movement reflected larger changes that were in the process of transforming American society. In the early twentieth century Progressive activists, whatever their
ideological persuasion, believed that the United States stood on the threshold
of a new social and moral order. Disagreements, of course, were by no means
absent; the range of Progressive thinking was sufficiently broad to encompass
quite different approaches. Some Progressives believed that evil and pathological behavior flowed from the immoral environmental circumstances in which
individuals lived; these reformers tended to favor interventionist measures designed to upgrade the circumstances in which people lived and worked. Others
were less sanguine about their ability to produce desired behavioral modifications simply by improving the environment. They supported coercive measures including, but not limited to, legislation that would exclude allegedly
"undesirable" immigrants, ban intoxicating liquors, and provide for the involuntary sterilization of "defective" persons. Whatever their ideological persuasion, Progressives shared a modern faith that the destiny of humanity could be
altered by conscious and purposive action.

The rise of industrialized society led many Progressives to favor national
action to deal with a variety of novel social and economic problems. Despite
differences in outlook, Theodore Roosevelt's New Nationalism and Woodrow
Wilson's New Freedom policies both envisaged a much more activist role for
the federal government. Although the Progressive movement of the early twentieth century and World War I also increased federal authority, the most significant catalyst of change was the Great Depression of the 1930s. During that
decade the economy was in shambles, millions were out of work, and most
state governments faced bankruptcy. The unprecedented economic crisis created a need to act as a nation rather than as a collection of semiautonomous
states. The election of Franklin D. Roosevelt in 1932 and his New Deal led to a
dramatic expansion in the role of the federal government as well as a new kind
of federalism. During the 1930s landmark legislation—notably the Social Security Act—set the scene for subsequent programs that transformed the lives of
millions of Americans. That serious (if unsuccessful) consideration was given

to national health insurance in that legislation was further evidence of the political transformation that was under way. Indeed, in subsequent decades the Social Security system was expanded to include disability insurance and medical coverage for the elderly, disabled, and indigent. All of these programs were to have a dramatic impact upon the lives of persons with serious and persistent mental disorders.

The New Deal was followed by World War II. During that conflict federal authority expanded in ways that affected the lives of virtually all Americans, whether in raising an army, placing the economy on a wartime footing, or imposing wage and price controls and instituting rationing. After the war some ultimately sought to expand federal responsibilities in health-related matters still further.

Undoubtedly the most important development in the last half century affecting those with serious mental illnesses has been the entrance of the federal government into the mental health policy arena. For better or worse, the fate of such persons has been shaped by a variety of federal programs. Some have represented specific choices; others were the result of a serendipitous process; and still others grew out of the peculiar structure of American government in which intergovernmental relations and rivalries played decisive roles. The emergence of the federal government as the major force in mental health policy shattered the traditional faith in institutional care and treatment. By the 1960s the legitimacy of mental hospitals was in question. Psychiatric activists and their allies promoted new policies designed to move care and treatment from hospitals to the community. At the same time they insisted that it was possible to identify individuals who were at high risk and for whom preventive therapies would eliminate or reduce the development of severe disorders. The result was a huge expansion of psychiatric diagnoses as well as mental health personnel. The assumption was that all of these changes would flow from enlightened federal leadership. Yet the outcomes of the vast changes in the mental health system were hardly those anticipated by their advocates. Indeed, in recent decades there has been a pronounced shift away from radical to incremental policy changes.

History, of course, never quite repeats itself, nor are its "lessons" self-evident. Nevertheless, we live with the results of the earlier policies. To be sure, much has changed, yet we continue to hear the same dissatisfactions and laments. If we are to develop strategies to mitigate the problems faced by persons with severe mental disorders, an understanding of the manner in which the federal government became a major force in mental health policy, the federal impact upon intergovernmental relationships, and the consequences of federal innovations is indispensable. Once created, policies and institutions acquire an independent existence that is not easily removed. Knowledge of their origins and development will not necessarily provide easy answers to difficult problems, but at the very least it will assist in developing a perspective that will avoid simplistic and unrealistic solutions. In the following pages we will both describe and analyze the profound changes in mental health policy since World War II and offer as well some personal observations.[18]

Chapter 1

Winds of Change

In 1945 the mental health establishment appeared stable; few observers questioned the presumption that the mental hospital was the proper place to provide care and treatment for persons with severe mental disorders. At that time the average daily resident population in public institutions was about 430,000; approximately 85,000 were first-time admissions. Nearly 88 percent of all patient care episodes occurred in these institutions; the remainder in general hospital psychiatric units.[1] In 1951 total state expenditures for all current operations were $5 billion. Of this sum, 8 percent was for mental hospitals. New York State spent no less than 33 percent of its operating budget on mental health; other states expended as little as 2 percent. Correspondingly, American psychiatry remained an institutional specialty; more than two-thirds of the members of the American Psychiatric Association (APA) practiced in public mental hospitals as late as 1940.[2]

The apparent stability of the mental health system, however, proved ephemeral. In the years following the end of World War II mental hospitals began to be perceived as the vestigial remnant of a bygone age. That they had failed to live up to their early promise was obvious. Their numerous problems—crowding, deteriorating physical plants, inadequately trained staffs, therapeutic shortcomings, and dehumanizing qualities—created an aura of profound disillusionment. Advocates for change urged that mental hospitals be replaced by new institutions that would treat individuals with severe mental disorders in the community. The emphasis on community care and treatment gave rise to what subsequently became known as deinstitutionalization. The fall in inpatient populations was striking. Between 1955 and 2000 the number of patients in American public mental hospitals declined from a high of 558,000 to 55,000.[3] The decline was even more dramatic if general population growth is taken into account. Had the proportion remained stable and the mix constant, mental hospitals would have had about 950,000 patients in 2000.

The origins of the policy of deinstitutionalization were anything but simple. A variety of factors played a role in creating alternatives to institutional care of persons with mental illnesses: humanistic and egalitarian ideologies that were common after World War II (in part a response to the perceived war against totalitarian regimes); the emphasis on the paramount role of environment in the social and behavioral sciences; the rise of psychodynamic psychiatry and its preoccupation with psychological factors in the etiology of mental disorders; the emergence of a literature that was critical of mental hospitals (as well as of other institutions) and their dehumanizing impact upon individuals; the spiraling costs associated with improved hospital care; and radical critiques of capitalist societies. Yet unique circumstances also created significant differences in the manner and timing in which deinstitutionalization was implemented in different states and regions.

The consequences of deinstitutionalization were equally complex. The decline in long-term hospitalization did not necessarily improve the lives of those intended as its beneficiaries. Ironically, the intent of deinstitutionalization as a policy has not always been clear. Indeed, over time it came to imply quite different meanings. In its origin, at least in the United States, it was synonymous with the creation of a linked and integrated system of services that would follow patients from the hospital into the community. Subsequently it implied the end of institutional care. More recently deinstitutionalization has referred to barriers to long-term inpatient residence. Whatever the meaning of deinstitutionalization, however, there is little doubt that outcomes have had relatively little to do with original intentions and expectations. Although not necessarily a complete failure, deinstitutionalization can hardly be characterized as a policy triumph.

In 1945 there was little evidence that the mental health scene would begin to undergo radical changes. Yet within a short time mental hospitals began to lose their social and medical legitimacy as the prevailing consensus on mental health policy dissolved. The experiences of the military during the war in successfully treating soldiers manifesting psychiatric symptoms and returning them to their units created a faith that outpatient treatment in the community would be more effective than confinement in remote institutions that shattered established social relationships. The war also hastened the emergence of psychodynamic and psychoanalytic psychiatry with its emphasis on the importance of life experiences and socioenvironmental factors. After 1945 many psychiatrists who had served in the military returned to civilian life determined to transform their specialty. Competing visions of the specialty were reflected in a struggle in the late 1940s within the APA. Those who had few links with mental hospitals and who were committed to psychodynamic and psychoanalytic theories, the significance of the social environment, social activism in a community setting, and various psychotherapies emerged triumphant. They would play a major role in reorienting mental health policy in succeeding years.[4]

From the mid-1940s to the 1960s the belief that early intervention in the community would be effective in preventing subsequent hospitalization and thus avoiding chronicity became an article of faith shared by many. As early as 1945 Robert H. Felix, an individual who played a major role in postwar mental health policy, argued that psychiatry had an obligation to "go out and find the people who need help—and that means, in their local communities." Three years later he and R. V. Bowers insisted that mental hygiene had to be concerned "with more than the psychoses and with more than hospitalized mental illness." Personality, after all, was shaped by socioenvironmental influences, and Felix and Bowers alluded to wartime psychiatric experiences. Psychiatry, in collaboration with the social sciences, had to emphasize the problems of the "ambulatory ill and the preambulatory ill (those whose probability of breakdown is high)." The community, not the hospital, was psychiatry's natural habitat.[5]

During the 1940s numerous critical accounts that detailed tragic conditions in mental hospitals began to appear. Journalists, notably Albert Deutsch, Albert Q. Maisel, and Mike Gorman, published devastating exposés. Deutsch's articles appeared in *PM* (a liberal New York City newspaper) in 1946 and 1947, and were followed by the publication the next year of *The Shame of the States*. Gaining national attention, the book was given added legitimacy by the inclusion of an introduction by Karl A. Menninger, a major figure in American psychiatry. Intended neither to discredit nor to undermine the legitimacy of mental hospitals, *The Shame of the States* was a clarion call for reform. At the same time *Life*—a magazine that reached an extraordinarily large and diverse audience—published Maisel's lengthy piece "Bedlam 1946." Its use of dramatic and horrifying photographs only added to its emotional impact. Gorman, a fledgling Oklahoma reporter, expanded a series of articles published in the *Daily Oklahoman* into a long article that appeared in *Reader's Digest*, a magazine read by millions of Americans. Unlike Deutsch and Maisel, Gorman was less concerned with reforming mental hospitals; he clearly favored a policy of early treatment in community settings. The most dramatic portrayal of the depths to which mental hospitals had allegedly fallen, however, came from the pen of Mary Jane Ward. Her novel *The Snake Pit*, published in 1946, serialized in *Reader's Digest,* and made into a film in 1949, depicted both severe institutional defects and the promise of psychodynamic and psychoanalytic psychiatry.[6]

During these same years psychiatrists were abandoning mental hospital employment for private and community practice. By the mid-1950s more than 80 percent of the 10,000 members of the APA were employed outside of mental hospitals. Institutional positions were increasingly filled by foreign medical graduates with little or no training in psychiatry.[7] Although the APA staff continued to work with public hospitals (especially through its Central Inspection Board, annual Mental Hospital Institutes, and by conducting surveys in individual states), most of its members were neither knowledgeable about nor sympathetic toward their institutional brethren and generally emphasized the desirability of noninstitutional alternatives. Psychiatrists in the community treated individuals with psychological problems and had relatively little contact with persons with severe and persistent mental illnesses.

That hospitals had a large proportion of long-stay patients with severe mental disorders hardly accorded with the self-image of psychiatrists as active and successful therapists. Indeed, in his APA presidential address in 1958, Harry C. Solomon—a distinguished figure in the specialty—even went so far as to describe the large public mental hospital as "antiquated, outmoded, and rapidly becoming obsolete." Robert C. Hunt, director of the Hudson River State Hospital in New York and an individual deeply concerned with institutional problems, responded publicly in critical terms. My "private reactions are still unprintable," he wrote to Solomon in angry words. Hunt subsequently informed the APA Commission on Long Term Planning that the organization had not played a constructive role in countering the detrimental effects associated with "the state hospital stereotype." The majority of APA members, he added, had neither contacts with nor knowledge about mental hospitals. Hence they were prone to conflate the prevailing stereotype with reality; the result was that the specialty had virtually abandoned a half million hospitalized patients.[8]

The dissolution of the traditional consensus on mental health policy, however, did not necessarily imply policy changes. The decentralized character of the American political system posed a barrier to broad policy change, since authority was vested in no less than forty-eight jurisdictions. That some would turn to the federal government as an agent of change was understandable, given federal prestige in the postwar years.

At this time strategically placed individuals and small groups had the ability to play prominent roles in federal policymaking. The relative insignificance of interest groups representing constituencies based on gender, race, class, and ethnicity only served to magnify their influence. Their efforts resulted in the passage of such landmark pieces of legislation as the Hill-Burton Act, which provided generous federal subsidies for hospital construction that added tens of thousands of new beds within a short period. At the same time the National Institutes of Health (NIH) was beginning its phenomenal expansion, thus making the federal government the major supporter of biomedical research and training and sharply reducing the importance of those philanthropic foundations that had been the main source of funding prior to 1940. These and other developments were furthered by close collaboration between federal officials such as Surgeon General Thomas Parran, public figures such as Mary Lasker, and key congressional allies.

That the public was receptive to such federal initiatives was clear. Faith in the redemptive powers of science, medicine, and technology had been spurred by such innovations as antibiotic therapy and the potential of unlimited atomic energy. The deliberations of President Harry S Truman's Scientific Research Board reflected the optimism of these years. Scientific discovery, insisted its members, was "the basis for our progress against poverty and disease." The board devoted an entire volume to medical research and the need for a "national policy." "The challenge of our times," wrote its members, "is to advance as rapidly as possible the understanding of diseases that still resist the skills of science, to find new and better ways of dealing with diseases for which some therapies are known, and to put this new knowledge effectively to work."[9]

Nowhere was the ability of individuals to influence policy better illustrated than in the passage of the National Mental Health Act of 1946. At that time there was as yet little interest in involving the federal government in mental health policy, which remained a responsibility of state governments. A Division of Mental Hygiene had been created within the Public Health Service (PHS) in 1930, but it dealt largely with narcotic addiction. In the late 1930s the psychiatrist Lawrence Kolb, its head, led an effort to create a National Neuropsychiatric

Institute modeled in part after the National Cancer Institute, which had been established in 1937. The initiative, however, failed as war-related concerns overwhelmed domestic issues.[10]

The task of integrating mental health within the burgeoning federal biomedical policy role was undertaken by Robert H. Felix, who had succeeded Kolb as head of the Division of Mental Hygiene in late 1944. Felix had received both his undergraduate and his medical degrees from the University of Colorado, and had worked under Franklin G. Ebaugh, an early proponent of the belief that individuals with mental disorders should receive treatment in general hospitals and thus avoid prolonged confinement in state institutions.[11] After spending eight years at several federal facilities, he was assigned to the Johns Hopkins University for training in public health. This experience had a profound impact on his understanding of psychiatry. Taking a public health approach, Felix became convinced that knowledge of the epidemiology of mental illnesses was crucial and that the social and behavioral sciences had much to contribute to an understanding of mental pathology.

Shortly after arriving at the Division of Mental Hygiene, Felix was urged by Surgeon General Parran to think about new responsibilities for the division. Felix then resurrected the Kolb proposal, but in sharply modified form. Kolb had been primarily concerned with research. Felix was by no means opposed to research. His agenda, however, was to expand the role of the federal government substantially and to use its authority to move away from an institutional toward a community-based policy. With the support of Parran and several figures at the Federal Security Agency (predecessor of the Department of Health, Education and Welfare), Felix drafted legislation creating a National Psychiatric Institute. A shrewd and charismatic individual, he proved a master of bureaucratic and organizational politics who cultivated close relationships with members of Congress in part through his willingness to provide them with assistance in coping with family members who had psychiatric problems. His draft of the legislation was characteristic. Its broad—even vague—provisions gave him the freedom to move in the direction he thought appropriate. Equally important, he believed that basic policy changes were a necessity. Yet he rarely concerned himself with details. The bill was introduced in Congress in the spring of 1945. After extended hearings in both chambers, the bill passed with virtually no opposition and was signed into law by President Truman on July 3, 1946.[12]

At that time there was little recognition that the National Mental Health Act of 1946 was a harbinger of things to come or that it represented the beginnings of a fundamental shift in the manner in which the nation dealt with severe mental disorders. The act provided for federal funding for research and training and authorized grants to states to assist them in establishing clinics, treatment centers, and demonstration projects. It also created two entities. A National Mental Health Advisory Council was given the responsibility of providing advice and recommending grants. More important, the act created the National Institute of Mental Health (NIMH), which became the second institute within the NIH. Under the leadership of Felix, its director from its formal creation in 1949 to 1964, the NIMH labored assiduously if quietly to create community-based institutions that would eventually replace mental hospitals. The legislation subtly began the process of transforming intergovernmental relationships by shifting authority to the federal government and eventually making it the major arbiter of mental health policy.[13]

The significance of the National Mental Health Act lay not in its specific provisions, but rather in its general goals and, more important, the manner in which it was interpreted and implemented. Indeed, federal policy in succeeding decades was often shaped less by congressional mandates and appropriations than by the outlook and actions of government officials charged with the responsibility for administering programs, writing regulations, and distributing funds. Congressional acts are often general in nature. Before becoming effective, they require administrative guidelines, and the preparation of such guidelines lies in the hands of federal officials employed in the executive branch of government. The role of these officials had been crucial, albeit unrecognized and unappreciated. Moreover, they have often used their close relationships with influential members of Congress to secure legislation that embody their policy goals.

By the time he had become NIMH director, Felix's views about the proper shape of mental health policy had matured. Although he remained friendly with both psychodynamic and somatic psychiatrists, he was never identified with either group. His underlying belief was that mental disorders represented "a true public health problem," the resolution of which required knowledge about the etiology and nature of mental illnesses, more effective methods of prevention and treatment, and better-trained personnel. Felix shared many of the views of Paul V. Lemkau of Johns Hopkins, an able and influential proponent of a public health approach and author of an important text on the subject. Public health, according to Felix, was concerned with the "collective health" of the community. Unlike clinicians who dealt with individuals, public health workers emphasized "the application and development of methods of mass approach to health problems," including mental illnesses. The NIMH program was designed "to help the individual by helping the community; to make mental health a part of the community's total health program, to the end that all individuals will have greater assurance of an emotionally and physically healthy and satisfying life for themselves and their families."[14]

Felix's agenda required radical changes in the prevailing institutional policy; he did not believe that an incremental approach could resolve problems. His goal was evident in the manner in which he interpreted the National Mental Health Act. In testimony before a congressional subcommittee in 1948, he maintained that the act precluded the use of federal funds for the support of hospitalization in state institutions. Such funds were rather to be used by states to create clinics and other alternatives to institutionalization. The ideal was to have one outpatient mental health clinic for each 100,000 people; rural areas would be served by traveling clinics. Moreover, it was evident that Felix's vision went far beyond individuals with severe mental illnesses. He told the subcommittee that if the "mentally ill" included the "emotionally disturbed" as well as those requiring "counseling or guidance or advice," the total would be around 8 to 10 million persons. The implication was clear; mental health required the infusion of vast sums of money.[15]

Felix's approach reflected his lack of clinical experience in dealing with persons with severe and persistent mental illnesses. Hence he favored a broad public health ideology. Only the "reintegration of community life" offered the possibility of reducing the incidence of mental disorders. Hostile to mental hospitals, he preferred large numbers of outpatient community clinics. Such institutions would avoid the stigmatization associated with mental hospitals and point the way to effective preventive programs. Indeed, the "guiding philosophy" of the NIMH, he told his APA colleagues in 1949, was that "the prevention of mental illness, and the production of positive mental health," was an "attainable goal."[16]

Cognizant that his policy goals were not achievable in the near future, Felix labored to make the NIMH a force in the mental health arena. A shrewd bureaucrat, he persuaded the surgeon general to place the NIMH within the NIH rather than under the Bureau of State Services, thus linking his organization with other research-oriented entities such as the National Cancer Institute. That the NIMH was indirectly involved in funding services as well as research and training was largely ignored. Indeed, demonstration clinics were placed under the rubric of research. In so doing Felix was able to exploit the identification of mental health with biomedical science during the 1950s.[17]

From the very beginning Felix and the NIMH undertook a variety of innovative activities designed to demonstrate that there were more effective ways of fostering mental health and diminishing the incidence of mental disorders. These ways included assistance to states by subsidizing the creation of clinics, the inclusion of the behavioral sciences and nonmedical personnel in mental health activities, and the awarding of research grants. The NIMH provided grants-in-aid to states to assist them in establishing and improving their mental health services. By 1947 every state and territory had designated an agency to prepare plans detailing the use of federal funds and to maintain liaison with the NIMH. Although funds could be used for a variety of purposes, federal officials encouraged states to develop additions, if not alternatives, to traditional mental hospitals.[18] The most significant impact of the state assistance program, however, was in the relationships that developed between the NIMH and health professionals employed in community institutions. The result was the creation of a new professional constituency that grew by leaps and bounds during the second half of the twentieth century. Its members would contribute to the effort to shift mental health services from state hospitals to community institutions, thus creating a potential conflict with their hospital brethren.

By the early 1950s changes in outlook and administrative practices were already beginning to modify traditional mental hospitals. After World War II Karl and William Menninger, in collaboration with state and federal authorities, transformed both Winter Veterans Administration Hospital and Topeka State Hospital in Kansas in a manner that suggested a greater therapeutic role. Two Massachusetts institutions, Worcester State Hospital and Boston Psychopathic Hospital, and Butler Health Center in Providence, Rhode Island, introduced changes that antedated the introduction of psychotropic drugs. Release rates at these institutions rose and average length of stays declined.[19]

Milieu therapy—the concept that environmental modifications within the mental hospital could be employed as a therapeutic tool—had been given concrete form by Maxwell Jones, a British psychiatrist who had worked with psychologically impaired servicemen and repatriated prisoners of war. Popularized in the United States by such figures as Alfred Stanton and Morris Schwartz, Milton Greenblatt, and Robert N. Rapoport, milieu therapy assumed that mental hospitals had an important role to play in providing care and active treatment.[20] At the same time the Council of State Governments (representing the nation's governors) and the Milbank Memorial Fund sponsored studies that emphasized the potential importance of community institutions.[21]

To institutional innovations was added the introduction of drugs, notably chlorpromazine, which ultimately reshaped psychiatric practice. The development of new pharmacological agents for the treatment of severe mental disorders was partly the result of chance, although Louis Pasteur's famous observation that "chance favors the prepared mind" is perhaps more accurate. In the 1940s clinical interest in the life-threatening effects of traumatic and surgical shock was widespread because of the experience with battlefield casualties in World War II. In 1949 Henri Laborit, who was seeking a means of preventing shock by inhibiting the autonomic nervous system, found that promethazine induced a "euphoric quietude" in surgical patients. The following year chlorpromazine was synthesized in France and was followed by a broad clinical study of its possible therapeutic effects in a variety of specialties. By 1952 it had been administered to individuals with severe mental disorders, with dramatic results. In the United States, Smith Kline & French began to market chlorpromazine as Thorazine. Shortly thereafter other major and minor tranquilizing drugs and antidepressants made their appearance, and slowly began to transform psychiatric practice.[22]

The institutional and therapeutic innovations of the 1950s seemed to presage a policy capable of realizing the dream of providing quality care and effective treatments for persons with mental illnesses. The simultaneous development of milieu therapy and the deployment of the new psychotropic drugs indicated a quite specific direction. Drug therapy would make patients amenable to milieu therapy; a more humane institutional environment would facilitate the release of large numbers of patients into the community; and an extensive network of local services would in turn assist the reintegration of patients into society and oversee, if necessary, their varied medical, economic, occupational, and social needs.

The innovations of this decade—both perceived and real—led some states to introduce institutional innovations. In 1954 New York enacted its influential Community Mental Health Services Act, which provided state funding for outpatient clinics. California followed suit shortly thereafter with the passage of the Short-Doyle Act. By 1959 there were more than 1,400 clinics serving slightly over a half million individuals, of whom 294,000 were over the age of eighteen.[23] The expansion of community facilities was also accompanied by new services to schools, courts, and social agencies provided by nonmedical mental health professionals. Slowly but surely the clientele of psychiatry and related disciplines expanded to include individuals other than those with severe mental illnesses.

Yet the policy debates of the 1950s manifested a curious ambivalence. Some believed that a linked and seamless integrated system that followed individuals from the hospital into the community represented the most desirable choice. Others looked forward to the day when traditional mental hospitals were replaced by institutions that offered care and treatment in the community. That there were similarities between them was clear; both accepted the ideology of community care and treatment. The former, however, believed that hospitals performed a vital role. If they were deficient, the remedy was to institute appropriate reforms. The latter, in contrast, insisted that hospitals were obsolete and should be eliminated over time. The conflict between those who favored incremental change and those who believed that only radical reform could alleviate problems was to be replicated throughout the remainder of the twentieth century.

In some ways the claims about the efficacy of community care and treatment rested on extraordinarily shaky foundations. The empirical data to support the claim that outpatient psychiatric clinics could identify early cases of mental disorders and also serve as alternatives to traditional mental hospitals were virtually nonexistent. Claims of accomplishment and effectiveness rested on ideology and faith, and were rarely, if ever, accompanied by empirical data. As early as 1950 a committee of the NIMH National Advisory Mental Health Council recommended that funds be allocated to develop methods "for determining the effectiveness of community mental health programs." Five years later council members expressed concern over "the vagueness surrounding the whole problem of community mental health." After surveying the literature, a subcommittee conceded that there was a "thinness of the efforts of evaluation" as well as a "confusion of levels of conceptualization."[24]

To be sure, the NIMH was not alone in heralding the importance of community mental health clinics and programs. During the 1950s, as well as in later decades, rhetoric rather than data often shaped policy discussions. The belief that many individuals—including those with severe and persistent mental illnesses—could be treated in outpatient clinics was an article of faith even though supporting data were largely absent. Indeed, data contradicting prevailing beliefs were all but ignored. In the mid-1950s a group of California researchers studied the effectiveness of hospital and clinic treatment in comparable psychiatric cases. The project involved three state hospitals and two state community clinics. From a sample of mental hospital admissions, the investigators screened 504 patients in the hope of referring them to clinics. Their experiences proved disheartening. Only 57 were identified as candidates for clinic referral; 20 of the 57 were referred; and 6 were accepted by clinics for treatment, of whom only 2 kept appointments and demonstrated any improvement. The investigators concluded that there were "marked discontinuities in functions" of hospitals and clinics. Individuals whose severe disorders created dependency and therefore required an extensive social support network were not candidates for clinics, which provided no assistance in finding living quarters or employment. In other words, the type of patients seen in clinics in general did not suffer from severe or persistent disorders; many were experiencing problems that accompanied the strains and stresses of everyday life. They were quite dissimilar from those admitted to hospitals. The investigators did not challenge the viability of clinics. Nevertheless, they suggested that the manner in which they were conceptualized required modification, and that far greater attention had to be paid to the development of links between clinics and hospitals.[25] Data collected by Morton Kramer and his colleagues at the Biometrics Branch of the NIMH raised equally serious problems. Three-quarters of institutionalized individuals had no families to provide care while undergoing rehabilitation in the community.[26]

The pace of change after 1945, however, seemed slow and unfocused. The NIMH was still in the early stages of growth. Nor had the federal government yet assumed a major policy role. The decentralized character of the American political system meant that the struggle to transform public policy had to be fought in each individual state. With forty-eight state legislatures and governors, the impediments facing the creation of a national policy seemed insuperable. Success was possible in large states such as New York and California, where concentrations of psychiatric personnel and services were present and public commitment to the welfare of persons with mental disorders was a long-standing tradition. In many states, however, different conditions prevailed and barriers to change were formidable.

The experiences of the New Deal, World War II, and the growing welfare role of the federal government, however, suggested a new direction for mental health policy. Psychiatric activists concluded that the time was ripe for a new initiative that would shift, at least in part, authority and responsibility in mental health from the states to the national government. The passage of the National Mental Health Act in 1946 had been an important first step. What was now required was legislation that redirected policy by providing generous federal funding. The passage of the Hill-Burton Act to subsidize hospital construction and growing federal support for biomedical research had already demonstrated the ability of the federal government to modify and reshape health policy. The existence of a biomedical lobby that included key congressional figures, a generalized faith in the ability of medical science to alleviate the burden of disease, and public receptivity to psychological explanations and interventions seemed to auger well for fundamental changes in mental health policy. To these was added a corresponding belief that many states were backward, parsimonious, and reactionary, whereas the federal government embodied wisdom, compassion, and generosity. The persistence of segregation and poverty as well as the absence of basic civil rights in many states only reinforced this general perception.

To shift policy authority from states to the federal government was a daunting task. In an effort to overcome impediments to change, psychiatric activists turned to the past for guidance. Their model was the famous report by Abraham Flexner for the Carnegie Foundation for the Advancement of Learning. Published in 1910, Flexner's *Medical Education in the United States and Canada* played a significant role in reforming medical education and laying a foundation for the subsequent preeminence of the United States in medical research and practice.[27] Why could not a comparable report on mental health policy ultimately lead to fundamental changes in the manner in which American society cared for persons with severe mental disorders?

The idea for a Flexner-type report was initially raised in 1953 by Kenneth E. Appel, then APA president and professor of psychiatry at the University of Pennsylvania. Two years later success came with the formal creation of the Joint Commission on Mental Illness and Health (JCMIH). There was unanimous agreement that the commission would be more effective if it were sponsored by professional organizations rather than by the federal government. The lead was taken by the APA and American Medical Association (AMA), which brought in representatives from the American Hospital Association, the Council of State Governments, the Veterans Administration, the NIMH, and other organizations representing nurses, psychiatric social workers, and clinical psychologists. In mid-1955 Congress passed the Mental Health Study Act. Under its provisions the federal government endorsed the creation of the JCMIH (which remained a nongovernmental body) and provided a modest level of funding to facilitate its work.[28]

Even though the JCMIH was dominated by mental health professionals, differences of opinion persisted. Should the commission focus on the problems of persons with severe mental disorders, or should it emphasize prevention and the promotion of mental health? Was it possible to study mental illnesses without an explicit concept of mental health? Were there important questions that could not be addressed simply because of the lack of knowledge or appropriate technologies? These were only a few of the complex issues that faced the JCMIH.

In the end participants adopted an agenda that was broad enough to conceal profound differences. First on the agenda was to study mental illness and health and the various "medical, psychological, social, cultural and other factors that relate to etiology." Second was to discover, develop, and apply appropriate methods for the diagnosis, treatment, care, and rehabilitation of persons with mental illnesses.[29] Third was to evaluate and to improve the recruitment and training of personnel. Fourth was to conduct a national survey of the problems posed by mental illness and mental health and to formulate a comprehensive program. The final item was to furnish to the federal and state governments as well as to the public the results of all the studies and surveys.[30]

The staff of the JCMIH conceded that underlying all of the processes of health lay a "biological stratum of organic and chemical factors." Nevertheless, their operational model emphasized the role of environment in the shaping of personality. At that time research on the physiological basis of mental disorders was extraordinarily difficult, if not impossible. Hence the commission relied largely on concepts common to psychodynamic psychiatry and the social and behavioral sciences, all of which were environmentally oriented. To create a knowledge base, a number of individuals were commissioned to prepare reports dealing with subjects such as manpower, patterns of patient care, the role of schools in the production of mental health, community resources in mental health, epidemiology, research, popular attitudes, economics, and concepts of mental health. Their work resulted in ten studies, nine of which were published in book form.[31]

That the authors of these studies did not always hold common views was evident. Yet the areas of agreement were striking. Most shared the belief that the pervasiveness of psychological and environmental stresses mandated an expansion of therapeutic services both within and without institutions; that early interventions would prevent the onset of more serious mental disorders; that the efficacy of social and psychological therapies was a matter of fact rather than a subject to be investigated; and that a concerted attack on the problems posed by psychological disturbances and mental illnesses required the creation of a broad coalition of professional and lay groups. Most significant, the thrust of their reports—though little noticed at the time—began to blur the distinction between individuals with problems, on the one hand, and persons with serious mental disorders, on the other. In ensuing policy debates, the central focus began to shift from the latter toward the former. The JCMIH did not consciously or deliberately downplay or ignore the problems faced by persons with serious mental illnesses. But those involved with the commission were beginning to expand, albeit slowly, the potential clientele of the mental health system, a shift that was not necessarily in the interests of those most in need of services.

By the summer of 1960 a draft of the final report was circulated to a JCMIH subcommittee for comment and advice. Its members were supportive of the view that mental health services were interdisciplinary in nature and that rivalries and competition over who was qualified to provide therapy were counterproductive. Some expressed concern that the draft "overemphasized . . . our knowledge of mental health" because of the need to increase research funding. In general, however, the discussion mirrored a broad consensus; differences were expressed only on marginal details.[32]

In March 1961 the final report of the JCMIH—*Action for Mental Health*—was transmitted to Congress and the nation's governors and released to the public with considerable fanfare. Written in lay rather than in medical or technical language, the document portrayed in dramatic terms the shortcomings of the mental health service system while at the same time sketching a vision for the future. The opening chapter cited the progress that had been made in providing facilities for care and treatment, but also emphasized that mental health programs lagged behind programs designed to treat other acute and chronic diseases.[33]

Therapeutic failures, the report noted, could not explain the lag in providing services. Indeed, the prognosis for functional psychoses was better than that of many malignancies. The basic problem was the failure of both the public and most of the medical profession to accept psychological illness as illness. People with severe mental illnesses aroused not sympathy but hostility. Madness broke the bonds that defined humanity and thus set its victims as a group apart. Consequently, public mental hospitals had evolved into dumping grounds for individuals beyond the pale of normal society.[34]

After summarizing the ten monographic studies and identifying issues and problems, *Action for Mental Health* recommended a comprehensive national program composed of four distinct but related elements. First, it called for a greater investment in basic research by allocating venture or risk capital to individuals, institutions, and the NIMH. Effective policies required that "the large gaps in our scientific knowledge about the fundamentals of mental illness and mental health" be diminished.[35]

Second, it offered recommendations relating to personnel and services that were designed to maximize the efficacy of existing knowledge and experience. It urged the adoption of a national recruitment and training program to increase the supply of trained personnel. To minimize jurisdictional rivalries among mental health disciplines it supported a "broad liberal philosophy" of treatment. Somatic therapies had to be provided by those with medical training. Psychoanalysis and "depth psychotherapy" had to be limited to physicians, psychologists, or other professionals with appropriate training and experience. Nonmedical workers, if qualified, could provide short-term psychotherapy. Since the demand for services would always exceed the supply, other occupational groups—teachers, clergy, social workers, family physicians, pediatricians, nurses, and others—could, with some training, assume the role of mental health counselors.[36]

In dealing with services, the report sketched out a program that was a reflection of postwar mental health ideology. Individuals with acute mental disorders required access to emergency care and treatment in both general and mental hospitals. The community mental health clinic, whether part of a general or mental hospital or a free-standing institution, was a main line of defense in reducing the need for prolonged and repeated hospitalization. Finally, general hospital psychiatric units would supplement clinic services.[37]

The report also included a radical and controversial recommendation, namely, that no state mental hospital with more than 1,000 beds be constructed, and that existing institutions with more than 1,000 beds be converted into centers "for the long-term and combined care of chronic diseases, including mental illness." In addition, aftercare and rehabilitation had to be integrated with all other services in order to minimize the need for hospitalization or rehospitalization.[38]

Third, *Action for Mental Health* identified a pressing need to disseminate information about mental disorders among the public in order to diminish stigmatization. Finally, the commission turned to the critical issue of financing. The basic problem, it insisted, was not economic but moral. "In conserving useful life, civilized man achieves his most glorious moments. It is our creed that life is sacred, that bodies should be healed when sick." What was required, therefore, was a doubling of public expenditures for public mental health services in five years and a tripling in ten. Such an ambitious goal could only be achieved by a massive increase in federal funding, which would be used as a lever to elevate standards of care and treatment. Reflecting the experiences of the New Deal and World War II, the individuals involved with the JCMIH believed that the federal government had both the resources and the wisdom to redirect mental health policy.[39]

Although a few members criticized some of the specific recommendations of the report, most were enthusiastic.[40] The document, of course, was not without ambiguity. Although emphasizing the importance of improving therapeutic and support services for persons with severe mental disorders, it also urged an expansion of services for troubled individuals who did not have a mental illness. These recommendations were not mutually exclusive, particularly in view of the claim that early treatment of the latter would diminish the incidence of serious mental disorders. But if the latter claim proved fallacious, the result might be the redirection of resources to serve troubled individuals. Under these circumstances individuals with severe disorders would suffer the consequences of having to compete for resources. In 1961 such concerns remained peripheral, and few could anticipate the outcome of policy innovations. *Action for Mental Health* was accompanied by a feeling of euphoria. If enacted into law, its recommendations, according to a press release, would "revolutionize public care of persons with major mental illness—the nearly 1,000,000 patients who pass through State hospitals and community mental health clinics each year."[41]

The case for change made by the JCMIH seemed compelling. Yet its final report was not a precise blueprint that could easily be translated into law; it merely suggested a general direction. What was required was the translation of broad goals and objectives into a specific legislative agenda that included adequate levels of funding. To move from advocacy to policy was by no means a simple task. In the larger political universe mental health advocates had to compete with a variety of other groups, each seeking support for their its program.

The creation of a political consensus on the need to reform the nation's mental health system faced a variety of obstacles. The goal of shifting more authority to the federal government was not universally accepted. Equally important, the reception of *Action for Mental Health*, though generally favorable, was by no means uncritical or one-sided. Given its global character, it would have been surprising if dissent had been absent.

Within the APA dissatisfaction with some of the recommendations of the JCMIH was evident. Some feared that psychiatric legitimacy and authority could be undermined by the use of mental health counselors. Discussions at more than half of the APA's district branches revealed concerns with the belief that psychotherapy and social therapy provided "answers to the prevention and cure of mental illness" and the ensuing disregard of the newer pharmacological and physical therapies. Nor was there agreement on the recommendation that the size of hospitals should be limited or expanded to include patients with other chronic illnesses. The most vociferous criticisms came from representatives of state hospitals, who believed that the commission overlooked the vital role of caring for and treating individuals with severe disorders—a group too often overlooked by psychiatrists in private practice. Similarly, a sample of the views of state commissioners of mental health found considerable ambivalence. After nine months of debate, the APA Council issued a generally laudatory position paper that offered support for many of the JCMIH recommendations. Nevertheless, its members expressed reservations. They thought that the 1,000-bed limitation was too arbitrary, nor did they agree with the proposal to convert large institutions into chronic care facilities. Indeed, they urged a continuation of efforts to upgrade rather than to transform the character of large state hospitals.[42]

The reaction of other organizations was similar. The AMA board of trustees resolved that *Action for Mental Health* was a "basis for a program." Its Council on Mental Health was supportive, although it reaffirmed its opposition to the practice of psychotherapy by nonmedical personnel. Ultimately the AMA adopted a program recommended by the Council on Mental Health that was disposed to retain local government fiscal responsibility. The board of directors of the American Psychological Association was generally favorable, but expressed criticism of the medical model of health and illness. Firm backing came from the National Association for Mental Health—the nation's foremost citizen's advocacy organization. Yet the organization omitted any mention of the proposal to transform large hospitals into chronic care institutions.[43]

State officials were not disposed to accept the JCMIH recommendations. A report from an Ad Hoc Committee on Planning for Mental Health Facilities, composed largely of these officials, did not envisage any fundamental changes in federal–state relations, but instead called for an expansion of community institutions within a state-planned, coordinated, and administered system. A special Governors' Conference on Mental Health in late 1961 adopted a policy statement that emphasized the need for community services, continuity of treatment, inpatient treatment in small mental hospitals, an expansion of general hospital psychiatric units, greater attention to research and training, and cost sharing between all levels of government.[44]

That there was no clear consensus on the recommendations of the JCMIH did not dampen the belief that some sort of action was required. The election of John F. Kennedy had created a favorable political climate, and public sentiment appeared supportive. The popularity of psychological theories and therapies had stimulated pressure for an expansion of psychiatric and psychological services. All of the elements for a new policy departure seemed in place; the remaining task was to tap into the massive financial resources of the federal government.

Critics of state social policymaking received indirect support from federal agencies, notably the NIMH. Felix and his colleagues were committed to a policy that both shifted the locus of care from hospitals to the community and provided services to the nonmentally ill. When asked to comment on a draft version of the final report of the JCMIH, Philip Sapir, chief of the Research Grants and Fellowship Branch, responded sharply that many statements were "pedestrian, platitudinous, rehashes of previous statements, half-truths, or untruths." Indeed, the draft was "so incredibly bad that there seems almost no point in making specific criticisms." His comments were echoed by Richard H. Williams of the Professional Services Branch of the NIMH.[45]

That those committed to new policies turned to the federal government was understandable. By this time there was a pervasive belief—not necessarily shared by all—that the national government was better qualified than its state counterparts to deal with pressing social problems. Indeed, the prevailing consensus was that most states had failed to meet their social welfare responsibilities. The tendency to denigrate state governments was also accompanied by an idealization of local communities and local control. This perception, which played an increasingly important role in the 1960s, tended to promote a vision of a federal–local government partnership that bypassed state authority not only in mental health but in other domestic welfare programs as well as in civil rights legislation.

The inauguration of President Kennedy in early 1961 and his call for a New Frontier raised the hopes of those who sought a new mental health policy departure. The Democratic Party platform had pledged federal support for research, training, and community mental health programs. Kennedy seemed favorably disposed, and his staff believed that the recommendations of the JCMIH could serve as the basis for "broadened Federal activity." But like his sister Eunice Kennedy Shriver, the president was concerned largely with retardation, subsequently redefined as "developmental disabilities." Indeed, in the view of those preoccupied with the fate of the retarded, *Action for Mental Health* was evidence of the lack of concern with this group. Nine months after taking office Kennedy created the President's Panel on Mental Retardation. Mental health, in contrast, had strong support in Congress. Faced with the prospect of political strife over priorities, Kennedy moved slowly in the months following his inauguration.[46]

In December Kennedy followed the advice of his staff and created an Interagency Task Force on Mental Health that included several high-level officials from the Department of Labor, the Veterans Administration, the Council of Economic Advisers, and the Bureau of the Budget. The real work, however, was done by a group of insiders that included Felix and his deputy, Stanley Yolles. Given Felix's stature, it was hardly surprising that he would play a dominant role in shaping the deliberations of the task force, many of whose members were willing to defer to professional authority.[47]

By this time the NIMH had prepared its own reaction to *Action for Mental Health*. It supported many of the recommendations, but disagreed that the care and treatment of persons with mental disorders was the core problem. Rather the commission should have focused more on "the prevention of mental illness and . . . maintenance of mental health." The NIMH rejected the recommendation that large state hospitals be converted into centers for the care of chronic patients and instead recommended the creation of a federal subsidy program to encourage states and communities to upgrade their activities in the prevention and treatment of mental illnesses.[48]

In the spring of 1962 two NIMH task forces had developed their own policy proposals. The first dealt with state hospitals. These institutions, insisted its members, reinforced "negative attitudes toward psychiatric treatment," fostered dependency, and were governed by an archaic administration. It urged that federal funds be used to assist states in developing new policies.[49]

The second task force, headed by Yolles, developed a comprehensive proposal that reflected a preference for a community-oriented public health approach. It expressed a faith in the efficacy of prevention and the effectiveness of community responsibility for the care, treatment, and rehabilitation of persons with mental disorders. If implemented, a community mental health program would make it possible "*for the mental hospital as it is now known to disappear from the scene within the next twenty-five years.*" Yolles and his colleagues then conceptualized a radically new institution, namely, a community health *center* (as compared with a clinic). The new center, they wrote, "is a multi-service community facility designed to provide early diagnosis and treatment of mental illness, both on an inpatient and outpatient basis, and serve as a locus for aftercare of discharged hospital patients." Centers would provide a broad spectrum of services: diagnosis and evaluation; inpatient care; day and night care programs; 24-hour emergency services; rehabilitation; consultive services to community agencies; public information and education; and supervision of foster care. They would serve designated populations within a defined geographical area. The task force envisaged a dramatic increase in federal funding and a major expansion in the role of the NIMH. In effect, the proposal suggested an entirely new policy direction that implied an eventual abandonment of institutional care.[50]

Although the Kennedy administration continued to express interest in mental health, it failed to develop a specific legislative agenda. Kennedy's reluctance to move was due in part to rivalry between mental health and mental retardation advocates. Pressure for action came from individuals such as Mike Gorman and William C. Menninger, as well as Lister Hill in the Senate and John Fogarty in the House of Representatives. The Committee on Appropriations, Fogarty noted in March 1962, "was disappointed that the budget did not include any plans for implementing the [JCMIH] Report. . . . The committee feels that the Executive Branch has been remiss in its duties in not yet having a plan for implementation before Congress."[51]

The following month Kennedy's interagency task force began its work in earnest. Influenced by and deferential to the views of Felix, its members agreed that the comprehensive community mental health center (CMHC) should become the basis for the president's policy. They accepted without question the claims that new knowledge about diagnosis, treatment, and prevention offered the potential for a new policy departure that "could really make a difference" and that state hospital populations could be reduced by half within a decade. To be sure, there were differences within the task force. Some believed that state control was obsolete and that an effective policy required increased federal funding and a measure of federal control. Others were hesitant about bypassing states and hoped that persuasion and education would suffice. A number of issues remained unresolved, including funding mechanisms and regulations. Nor did the group address the problem of staffing the projected number of centers or their impact upon intergovernmental relations. In the end members proposed a public health approach that they hoped would eliminate state mental hospitals within a generation. The goal was to create 500 centers by 1970 and an additional 1,500 a decade later. Federal grants would assist in their construction and gradually decreasing grants would cover initial operating expenses.[52]

That the interagency task force had ignored, if not rejected, the JCMIH recommendations was evident. Even more significant, however, was the absence of any evaluation of the claims that CMHCs could eliminate the need for institutional care within a generation. Ideology and assumptions rather than evidence became the basis on which new policy was formulated. Indeed, by the 1960s rhetorical claims about community superiority had created an irresistible momentum. Federal beneficence and wisdom, combined with community enlightenment would presumably create a new kind of institution that would overcome the myopic inability of states to pursue effective mental health policies. The task force thus developed a paradoxical synthesis that rationalized centralized control and local autonomy while implicitly bypassing and weakening the mediating role of state governments.

A discordant note sounded when Anthony Celebrezze, secretary of the Department of Health, Education and Welfare (DHEW) resisted the proposal that federal subsidies provide operating funds for centers. Faced with opposition, Celebrezze reversed himself and in the late autumn of 1962 submitted his recommendations to the White House. Public policy had to incorporate two objectives. The first included measures "to promote mental health and prevent mental illness." The second was an emphasis on cure rather than incarceration. The time had come "when almost all the mentally ill could be cared for in treatment centers in their own communities." These goals would be implemented by the creation of a "comprehensive community mental health center—a comparatively new concept which offers exciting possibilities for upgrading mental health services."[53]

The recommendations of the interagency task force and DHEW raised a series of important and controversial issues that required White House adjudication. There were, after all, fundamental differences between the JCMIH, on the one hand, and the task force and DHEW, on the other. The JCMIH had envisaged a far more significant role for the federal government. DHEW, in contrast, combined fiscal prudence with policy radicalism. Moreover, issues of feasibility remained unresolved. Were there sufficient qualified personnel to staff the proposed 2,000 CMHCs? It was doubtful that schools of nursing and social work had the capacity to meet projected needs. Equally significant, the goal of increasing the number of psychiatrists could only be met by dramatically reducing the supply of general practitioners and specialists, thus exacerbating other health problems.[54]

When the Panel on Mental Retardation offered its own recommendations in the autumn of 1962, the stage was set for some form of presidential decision.

In December mental health and mental retardation advocates met with officials from Kennedy's staff, the Bureau of the Budget, DHEW, the Public Health Service, and the Council of Economic Advisers. Subsequently Kennedy agreed to support a major federal initiative. Continued friction between mental health and mental retardation forces led the administration to support an omnibus bill that included both. Such a tactic, recalled Myer Feldman, a member of Kennedy's staff, made the program "more saleable."[55]

On February 5, 1963, Kennedy forwarded to Congress his message dealing with mental illness and retardation. His reputation as a champion of these disabled groups is somewhat inaccurate. When shown a draft of his message, he offered neither comments nor modifications and simply accepted it. This passivity was somewhat uncharacteristic, for his normal pattern was to make changes. In this instance he accepted Feldman's and Eunice Shriver's assurances that the substance and form of the message was appropriate. On retardation he deferred to his sister; on mental health he relied on his advisers.[56]

In his message Kennedy called for a "a bold new approach" that relied "primarily upon the new knowledge and new drugs . . . which make it possible for most of the mentally ill to be successfully and quickly treated in their own communities and returned to a useful place in society." For too long individuals with severe mental disorders had been confined within an "antiquated, vastly overcrowded, chain of custodial State institutions." A new mental health program could within a decade or more reduce the number of individuals under custodial care by 50 percent or more. What was required was a greater emphasis on the prevention of mental disorders and the training of personnel. The centerpiece of the new program was the comprehensive community mental health center. Kennedy recommended that the federal government provide funds to subsidize the construction of CMHCs. In addition, staffing grants limited to four years would assist such centers to begin operations.[57]

Although Kennedy's message received favorable national publicity, the barriers that impeded decisive action were formidable. Mental health and retardation had to compete with other administration health policy initiatives in a Congress that was increasingly wary of deepening federal involvement in such areas. Nor was the administration especially adept in dealing with the House and Senate, and several other major initiatives remained stalled. In addition, the NIH biomedical research programs, which previously had received enthusiastic congressional support, were coming under legislative scrutiny because of underlying managerial problems.

Fortunately for the administration, several key congressional figures came to its support. In the Senate Lister Hill, a long-standing proponent of federal activism in health policy issues who chaired the Committee on Labor and Public Welfare as well as the Committee on Appropriations, scheduled public hearings, thus inhibiting the emergence of an organized opposition. A litany of prominent individuals and organizational representatives from the mental health field extolled the virtues of CMHCs in glowing language. "I wish to God I could live and be active for 25 more years," stated Felix, "because I believe if I could, I would see the day when the State mental hospitals as we know them today would no longer exist, but would be a different kind of institution for a selected few patients who needed specialized types of care and treatment." Perhaps the most striking testimony was offered by Jack Ewalt, who had directed the JCMIH. The proposed legislation, he insisted, had grown out of the work of the commission. In point of fact, *Action for Mental Health* had been largely directed at the improvement of the care and treatment for those with severe mental disorders (though not ruling out additional services for non–mentally ill persons). The bill, in contrast, was designed to create a novel institution with a less clearly defined but global focus.[58]

In the House the bill came under much greater scrutiny during public hearings. When Celebrezze testified during a subcommittee hearing, he was so ineffectual that part of his presentation was excised from the printed record. Several committee members raised searching questions. Paul Rogers, a knowledgeable figure about health-related matters, expressed serious doubts about the feasibility of staffing of centers with qualified personnel. Some were concerned about growing federal involvement and the shift of authority from states to local communities. Others questioned the claim that subsidies for staffing were only temporary.[59]

Yet with some exceptions, the hearings in both chambers proved a rhetorical exercise; few legislators were willing to question professional authority. Indeed, a peculiar partnership of professional omniscience and political deference dominated the proceedings. There was no effort to evaluate claims that CMHCs could deal with the problems of persons with severe disorders. Nor was there any discussion about the difficulties of integrating former patients into society. Assertions about continuity of care and integration of services were thematic statements that did not address the formidable administrative and bureaucratic problems of implementing an effective community policy. Nor was there any discussion of the fate of the large numbers of elderly persons who were confined in mental hospitals. Ideology triumphed over reality and created a euphoric atmosphere conducive to favorable congressional action.

Even before the House hearings, Hill recognized the pitfalls that faced the legislation, particularly the provision providing federal support for staffing. He therefore persuaded the administration to support the merger of mental health and mental retardation into a single bill; the popularity of the latter might overcome opposition to the former. Opposition to the bill by the AMA House of Delegates led the House to delete the provision providing for federal subsidies for staffing. Fear that the legislation would fail if the Senate refused to concur, an amended bill without staffing finally passed and was signed into law on October 31 by President Kennedy.[60]

The mental health provisions of the Mental Retardation and Community Mental Health Centers Construction Act were relatively simple. It provided a three-year authorization for grants totaling $150 million for fiscal years 1965 through 1967 for construction; the federal share ranged between one-third and two-thirds. States were required to submit a comprehensive plan; designate an agency to administer the plan; create an advisory council with broad representation; and establish a construction program based on a statewide inventory of existing facilities and needs. The designated state agency would forward construction applications to Washington for final approval. The legislation, proclaimed Felix, reflected the concept that many forms of mental disorders could be "prevented or ameliorated more effectively through community oriented preventive, diagnostic, treatment, and rehabilitation services than through care in the traditional—and isolated—state mental hospital."[61]

Hailed as the harbinger of a new era, the act anticipated the creation of 2,000 CMHCs by 1980. Nevertheless, the creation of this novel institution was marked by paradox and ambiguity. The widespread assumption that public mental hospitals merely served warehousing and custodial functions and therefore deserved to be abandoned, for example, was somewhat overdrawn. Such institutions were not without major shortcomings, but such criticisms were exaggerated. Beginning in the 1950s Morton Kramer and his colleagues at the Biometrics Branch of the NIMH had begun to collect new kinds of data about the institutionalized population. They found that longitudinal data revealed the length of stay for individuals diagnosed with schizophrenia had been declining for thirty years. In 1948, for example, 56 percent of such cases were discharged within twelve months, as compared with only 33 percent in 1914. In the same period the number of resident patients suffering from the physical and mental infirmity of old age had risen from 24 to 42 percent. In other words, mental

hospitals were caring for ever larger numbers of elderly patients because of declining mortality rates. For many of these individuals some sort of institutional
care was a necessity. The abolition of mental hospitals would not resolve the
difficult task of providing care for these aged and dependent individuals.

Other data raised equally serious questions. A community policy was
based on the expectation that patients could be treated in noninstitutional settings. Underlying this belief were several assumptions. First, that patients had
a home. Second, that patients had a sympathetic and supportive family or care-
giver willing and able to assume responsibility for their well-being. Third, that
the organization of the household would not impede rehabilitation. Fourth,
that the patient's presence would not cause undue hardships for other family
members. Finally, that social support networks and occupational opportunities
were available. In point of fact, few of these assumptions reflected reality. In
1960, 48 percent of the mental hospital population were unmarried, 12 percent
were widowed, and 13 percent were divorced or separated. In other words, the
majority of patients might have no families to care for them. The claim that
persons with severe mental disorders could reside in the community while
undergoing rehabilitation was hardly realistic, given the fact that no provision
whatsoever had been made to provide a network of social support structures
and housing.[62]

When the JCMIH was created in 1955, the central concern was with persons with severe mental illnesses and especially those who were institutionalized. Eight years later Congress enacted a law that dramatically shifted the
focus to an institution that represented a radical policy break. In place of a
program of incremental change, it chose instead to embark on a new beginning
that would sweep away the legacy of a dismal past. What had begun as an effort
to improve the lot of a dependent population concluded with the creation of a
novel institution.

The new departure had major implications for the pattern of intergovernmental relations. Historically, health services were under the jurisdiction of
state and local governments. Even as the federal role in health policy increased
after 1945, it rarely included direct services. Instead the national government
focused on subsidies for hospital construction (Hill-Burton) and the support
of biomedical research. The act of 1963, by contrast, differed in fundamental
respects. In effect, the federal government undertook to reshape policy by forging direct links with local communities. Such an administrative procedure
heightened the policymaking role of professionals and federal officials, few of
whom had direct links with mental hospitals. The function of state authorities

was relegated to forwarding construction applications conceived and developed at the local level as part of a comprehensive plan to regionalize mental health services.[63]

Aside from the consequences for intergovernmental relationships, the act of 1963 created an institution whose nature and functions were unclear and whose potential clientele was protean and not limited to persons with severe and persistent mental disorders. No effort was made to spell out the relationships between CMHCs and mental hospitals, nor was serious consideration given to the ways in which centers would or could assume the caring roles of hospitals. Moreover, the provisions of the legislation gave DHEW responsibility for defining the essential services of centers. After a bureaucratic struggle, Felix had the program placed within the NIMH rather than the Bureau of Medical Services, which had responsibility for overseeing hospital construction under the Hill-Burton Act. By early 1964 NIMH officials issued regulations that defined five essential services that CMHCs were required to provide: inpatient services; outpatient services; partial hospitalization services, 24-hour emergency services within the three previous services; and consultation and educational for community agencies and professional personnel. The most curious aspect of the regulations was the omission of any mention of state hospitals. In one sense this was understandable, given the belief that centers would replace hospitals. Nevertheless, the absence of linkages was striking. If CMHCs were designed to provide comprehensive services and continuity of care, how could they function if they were isolated from the nearly half million hospitalized patients? Indeed, the absence of linkages facilitated the development of a system of centers that ultimately catered to a quite different population and largely ignored the needs of persons with serious mental disorders. On several other issues the regulations remained silent. They did not identify the professional group that would have primary responsibility for administering centers, although psychiatrists were to control the clinical program. Nor did the regulations (or, for that matter, the legislation) define the meaning of *community*. Since Felix and his colleagues found that political, geographical, ethnic, or socioeconomic boundaries did not work, they fell back on numbers. They defined a community by stipulating a population range of 75,000 to 200,000.[64]

State hospitals were not entirely ignored. The Hospital Improvement Program, proposed by the NIMH and modestly funded by a sympathetic Congress in 1964, presumably provided resources to enable hospitals to plan a transitional mission until their functions could be assumed by the new centers.

Under the program, however, grants to hospitals were limited to $100,000 per year. Planners, charged two psychiatrists employed by the state of Illinois, were "operating on the assumption that state hospitals cannot be significantly improved and that imposing the new model of the community mental health center will obviate the need for state hospitals." The result, they added, would be to create "two worlds of mental health care." The CMHC would "become a showcase, treating selected patients," whereas the majority of those needing services would be relegated to mental hospitals, receiving "only a small fraction of the treatment resources."[65]

The final element in the new community-oriented system—legislation providing for federal support for staffing centers—was put into place in 1965. The accession of Lyndon Johnson to the presidency in late 1963 and his overwhelming victory over Barry Goldwater in the election of 1964 had brought to the White House a shrewd, determined, forceful, and sometimes ruthless individual determined to push his Great Society program. Within this context the NIMH renewed its support for the staffing bill. Admittedly, dissatisfaction within the mental health constituency was present. State officials such as Dr. David Vail of Minnesota insisted that centers could not alleviate "social ills," and he called for measures to strengthen the state hospital system and to fill gaps at the community level. Others were critical of the effort to bypass state authority and insisted that the center concept was poorly conceived. Nevertheless, the strength of those who favored a community policy proved irresistible. The weakness of the AMA, which was preoccupied with the Medicare bill, spurred efforts to enact the staffing law. In mid-1965 legislation easily passed Congress authorizing grants for staffing CMHCs and providing new services. The subsequent regulations promulgated by the NIMH reflected once again the triumph of the ideology of community care. CMHCs were given responsibility for the "mental health of the community, . . . the prevention of mental illness and the more rapid and complete recovery of persons affected with mental illness in the community, . . . [and] the development of improved methods of treating and rehabilitating the mentally ill."[66]

The advocates of community care and treatment had spelled out a radical vision of change. They had created a novel institution—the CMHC—that would presumably diminish, if not eliminate, the traditional state hospital that had been at the center of mental health policy for nearly 150 years. Although details were lacking, supporters of CMHCs took for granted their ability to deal effectively with the problems faced by persons with severe mental disorders as well as by psychologically troubled individuals. The pervasive confidence during these years grew out of a conviction that medical and scientific advances, combined with novel institutional structures and enlightened federal leadership, provided the mechanisms that would create a new and more effective public policy. That the consequences of their actions would not always reflect their aspirations and expectations would only become apparent in years to come.

Chapter 2

Policy Fragmentation

By 1965 psychiatric activists believed that they stood on the threshold of a new era. In their eyes the passage of the CMHC act and the subsequent legislation providing for federal funding for staffing had created the foundation for fundamental changes in the mental health system. They anticipated that the new community-based policy would eventually lead to the disappearance of traditional mental hospitals. Moreover, they had faith that early identification and the deployment of appropriate interventions and caring systems as well as preventive measures would not only reduce the number of individuals at risk but also lead to dramatic improvements in the lives of those with serious and persistent mental disorders as well as those beset by psychological problems.

Community psychiatry—the term frequently employed in the 1960s—was heralded as the beginnings of a new psychiatric revolution. The new psychiatry, according Louis Linn, was designed to saturate "a given geographical area with medical services aimed at all levels of prevention and treatment for the families who reside therein." The community psychiatrist, wrote Gerald Caplan of the Harvard Medical School, was concerned not with the "individual peculiarities of a single patient, but [with] broad issues of mental disorder and its causation which apply to populations of patients." The goal was to develop "programs of intervention which will significantly affect many people not only by his direct intervention with them, but also indirectly through the mediation of other caregivers and by altering social and cultural influences which affect them." Caplan's popular *Principles of Preventive Psychiatry* symbolized the expansive claims that were so common during the 1960s.[1]

The growing role of the federal government and the enactment of legislation mandating new initiatives designed to remedy the shortcomings of the traditional institutional policy, however, did not ensure that the desired outcome would embody its original intent. Legislation generally assumes a static universe; a legal mandate supposedly alters individual and group behavior as well as institutional arrangements in ways that overcome older policy deficiencies. But reality is far more complex. Faced with laws designed to transform policy, individuals and groups often adjust their behavior in the light of new realities. In so doing they transform legislative intent in unforeseen and unpredictable ways, thus giving rise to unanticipated consequences. The history of mental health policy during these years vividly illustrates the validity of this generalization.

CMHCs, for example, assumed functions that were unanticipated by their promoters. The treatment of choice at most centers was individual psychotherapy, an intervention especially adapted to a middle-class educated clientele who did not have severe disorders and which was congenial as well to the professional staff. The result was that persons with severe and persistent mental disorders—the group with the greatest needs—were generally overlooked or else, forced to compete with other groups for resources, were often the losers.

The creation of CMHCs also occurred at a time in which social and political conflicts were accompanied by demands for civil rights and greater equality as well as criticisms of the growing American involvement in Vietnam. The antiorganizational ideologies that emphasized the importance of community activism by hitherto marginal groups led some CMHCs to devote their energies to improvement of social conditions. "The success of a mental health program," two NIMH officials remarked in an address at the American Psychopathological Association in early 1967, "is no longer simply a function of the clinical skills of the program staff; the success of a program is equally dependent on skills in coping with, and adapting to, and sometimes even changing the local political, social, and economic environment."[2] The focus of some CMHCs on social action only served to deflect their energies still further away from the needs of persons with serious disorders.

Nor were the unanticipated results of the CMHC legislation unique. When Lyndon B. Johnson took office following the assassination of President Kennedy and swept to an overwhelming victory in the election of 1964, he presided over a dramatic expansion of the social welfare role of the federal government. His Great Society program was designed not only to reduce poverty and expand civil rights but to provide health benefits for elderly, disabled, and indigent persons. Although designed for quite different purposes, landmark pieces of legislation such as Medicare and Medicaid assumed a critical role in reshaping the mental health system. Medicare and Medicaid, as well as other entitlements, had the inadvertent effect of hastening the deinstitutionalization of patients, but without ensuring the availability of comprehensive community services and structures.

The emphasis on social action and expansive claims that psychiatry and other mental health professions could be catalytic forces for social, economic, and cultural change that were so characteristic of these years mirrored a subtle political transformation. Groups that defined themselves in terms of race, gender, class, religion, and ethnicity were now changing part of the configuration of American politics. In many respects this transformation created the foundation for a sustained attack on discriminatory practices that had marginalized minorities, women, and individuals with disabilities, all of whom benefited to some degree. But it also altered in fundamental ways the policymaking process. From the 1940s to the 1960s strategically placed individuals and small groups played major roles in policy formulation. Federal bureaucrats such as Robert H. Felix and Mary Switzer, laypersons such as Mary Lasker, and a congressional health lobby that included Senator Lister Hill and Representative John Fogarty had the ability to influence and to shape health policy. By the 1970s a quite different situation prevailed. The proliferation of interest groups introduced a new element and gave policymaking a different character. The role of individual leadership was partially diminished. In the new political environment the absence of a group representing persons with severe disorders meant that their needs and interests would often be subordinated to better-organized groups.

Despite high hopes, the creation and construction of CMHCs moved at a slow pace. A significant element was the shortage of professional personnel. Equally important, appropriations for both construction and staffing fell far short of authorizations as costs of the Vietnam War mounted. The original legislation assumed that 2,000 CMHCs would be in existence by 1980; the actual number by that year was 754. Moreover, many of the centers were located in less urbanized areas. During the 1970s, for example, cities with populations between 10,000 and 50,000 accounted for 40 percent of the total. By then it had become abundantly clear that—whatever their actual functions—CMHCs were not serving as replacements for traditional public mental hospitals.[3]

Even if the goal of creating 2,000 centers had been met, it is not at all clear that they would have met the needs of persons with serious and persistent mental illnesses. At the very outset there was no consensus on the kinds of individuals that these institutions would serve. The often-advanced claim that it was possible to identify individuals who—if untreated—would be at high risk to become mentally ill had little if any foundation in fact. Much the same was true for claims about the efficacy of preventive programs. Nor did those involved in policy decisions pay attention to the behavior of consumers. In the postwar decades Americans became enthusiastic users of medical services, both regular and irregular. The belief that environmental and interpersonal relationships played major roles in creating psychological maladjustment only added to the pressure to provide mental health services for a broad public. Faith in the efficacy of medical science and employer-paid health insurance combined to alter traditional usage patterns. From their very beginnings CMHCs dealt largely with individuals who were experiencing problems in living rather than with those with serious mental disorders; psychotherapy was the major focus. Nor did centers provide coordinated aftercare services and continuing assistance to individuals who had been discharged from mental hospitals. Much the same was true of psychiatrists in private practice.[4]

The weaknesses of intergovernmental linkages and the increasing diversity and complexity of the mental health arena only exacerbated existing problems. During the 1960s faith in "community action"—whatever the meaning of that term—and the trend to bypass state regulatory agencies because of their alleged ineffectiveness left CMHCs free to move in directions that were not always conducive to meeting the needs of persons with severe mental disorders. According to prevailing attitudes, such individuals, after all, presented formidable problems. They were not easily managed; they generally required comprehensive care; they were poor candidates for psychotherapies; and their illnesses created dependency. Comprehensive services found in mental hospitals, however problematic, were not easily provided in community settings. Who would ensure that persons with severe and persistent mental illnesses would have access to housing, food, psychiatric care, social support systems, and occupational opportunities? To provide for the needs of such persons outside of institutions was daunting, and the available means of administration, rhetorical claims notwithstanding, were rarely equal to this task. Under such circumstances it was understandable that CMHCs were more responsive to local pressures to provide a variety of services for a quite different population that included individuals experiencing problems in living, children, and substance abusers (alcoholics, drug users). This is not to insist that centers completely ignored those with severe illnesses. In 1975, for example, 10 percent of their admissions were from the schizophrenic category.[5] But such data suggest how far they had deviated from the intent of those responsible for their founding.

The ever-growing role of the federal government and the NIMH only exacerbated friction with state authorities. At an NIMH-sponsored conference in 1966 a number of state representatives indicated their dissatisfaction. Public mental hospitals could not be ignored; many provided high-quality comprehensive services. CMHCs, they added, ought to be not freestanding, but rather part of an integrated service system. Despite these entreaties, CMHCs by and large followed an independent path in succeeding years. Moreover, there was a steady decline in the number of psychiatrists who either directed or were employed in centers. Between 1970 and 1981 the number of average full-time equivalent psychiatrists declined from 6.8 to 3.8, whereas the comparable figure for clinical psychologists rose from 4.9 to 9.4.[6]

Paradoxically, inpatient populations at state mental hospitals began a dramatic decline after 1965. Between 1955 and 1965 the inpatient population was reduced by about 15 percent, a relatively modest fall. In the succeeding decade, however, there was a fourfold increase in the decline (about 59 percent). Nevertheless, rates of deinstitutionalization were by no means uniform. Between 1967 and 1973 five states reduced their inpatient populations by 20 percent or less, twenty-two states by 21 to 40 percent, and five by 61 to 80 percent. The variability in rates was a natural consequence of differing traditions and conditions in individual states.[7]

The decline in inpatient mental hospital populations, however, had little to do with CMHCs, which were serving a quite different clientele. In urban areas in particular CMHC clients, as compared with inpatient mental hospital patients, tended to be younger, poorer, and disproportionately drawn from minority and nonwhite backgrounds. Many were referred to centers because of alcoholism and drug addiction, which by now were subsumed under mental health. Indeed, much of the testimony before various congressional committees considering the role of centers dealt with addiction. Believing that CMHCs had contributed to the fall in hospital populations, Congress enacted a series of laws expanding the responsibilities of centers to include the prevention and treatment of alcoholism and drug addiction.[8]

Nor was the decline in hospital populations after 1955 due—as many be-lieved—to the introduction of Thorazine in the mid-1950s in large state institu-tions. New medications were important in reducing the positive symptoms of psychosis and gave hope and confidence to the medical and supportive staff, administrators, and families that patients could be managed with fewer re-straints. However, there is evidence that the introduction of new pharmaceuti-cals was not sufficient to explain changes in patterns of care. In some localities deinstitutionalization preceded the introduction of new drugs. At Worcester State Hospital in Massachusetts, for example, a change in outlook and adminis-trative practices in the early 1950s hastened release rates back into the commu-nity. These changes, which occurred elsewhere at institutions such as Boston Psychopathic Hospital and the Butler Health Center in Providence, antedated the introduction of drugs. Moreover, the average length of stay declined as well. The introduction of drugs often facilitated a trend that was already transform-ing institutional practices.[9]

The greatest decline in inpatient populations occurred after 1965 and fol-lowed the enactment of far-reaching amendments to the Social Security Act of 1935. This landmark legislation, though best known for its old age assistance and insurance programs, included provisions dealing with health and wel-fare. Incremental changes altered and broadened the act in subsequent years. In 1956 amendments to the act created Social Security Disability Insurance (SSDI), which provided benefits to individuals fifty years and older who were unable to hold jobs because of their physical or mental condition. Four years later this age limitation was deleted. Although subsequent changes broadened the act's provisions, the most significant change came in 1965 with the creation of Medicare and Medicaid.[10] The most surprising feature of these amendments was the inclusion of psychiatric benefits.[11]

The enactment of Medicare and Medicaid seemingly had little to do with mental health policy. Yet both had a profound impact on mental hospital pop-ulations. Equally significant, they greatly expanded the federal role in mental health policy. Medicaid in particular became an important source of fund-ing for the care of elderly patients in mental hospitals. More important, both programs contributed to a shift in mental hospital populations. Between 1965 and 1972, for example, annual first admissions of individuals aged sixty-five or older fell from 26,606 to 14,490. Even more striking, the rate per 100,000 declined from 146 to 69. This is not to suggest that elderly individuals suffer-ing from a mental disorder or senility were no longer institutionalized. Instead the locus of care of these individuals shifted from mental hospitals to nursing homes. In 1964 nursing homes cared for over half a million people, of whom nearly 20 percent were diagnosed with a mental illness and just over a quarter as senile. By 1973 the entire nursing home population had doubled, and 25 percent were diagnosed with a mental illness and 58 percent as senile. What occurred in effect was a lateral shift. Aged as well as younger persons with a diagnosis of mental illness were sent in ever larger numbers to nursing homes rather than to state hospitals because of generous federal payments for care in nursing homes. By 1977, 14 percent of the total Medicaid funds spent on mental health supported elderly patients in state hospitals, and 53 percent supported elderly and nonelderly individuals in nursing homes. A study by the General Accounting Office (GAO) in 1977 noted that Medicaid was "one of the largest single purchasers of mental health care and the principal federal program funding the long-term care of the mentally disabled." It also was the most significant "federally sponsored program affecting deinstitutionaliza- tion." Yet the decline in state mental hospital populations was not necessarily synonymous with deinstitutionalization; it merely reflected a shift of indi- viduals from mental hospitals to chronic care nursing facilities. The driving force in this development was the ability of states to shift the costs of care to the federal government. In effect, Medicaid in particular provided states with an entrepreneurial opportunity that they seized with alacrity. The shift from mental hospital to nursing facility care was a development driven by a desire to promote the use of federal resources rather than by a desire to improve the lot of elderly persons and others with a severe and persistent mental disorder. Nor did this shift necessarily raise the quality of care. Indeed, the decentraliza- tion of institutional care (the substitution of nursing homes for mental hospi- tals) often exacerbated the problem of providing humane care, if only because of the difficulties of overseeing the thousands of nursing homes that had come into existence.[12]

In the 1970s the decline in mental hospital populations continued at a rapid pace as federal entitlement programs continued to play an ever more sig- nificant role. In 1972 the Social Security Act was further amended to provide coverage for individuals who had in the past not qualified for benefits. Under the provisions of Supplemental Security Income for the Aged, the Disabled, and the Blind (more popularly known as SSI), all those whose age or disability rendered them incapable of holding a job became eligible for income support. Administered and funded by the federal government, these Social Security en- titlement programs had the added virtue of minimizing the stigmatization often associated with welfare. SSI and SSDI hastened the discharge of patients from mental hospitals, since federal payments would enable them to live in the community. Moreover, they became eligible for Medicaid coverage, housing supports, and food stamps, thus adding to the resources available to them.

The expansion of federal entitlement programs was the driving force behind the decline in mental hospital populations during the 1970s and after, a trend reflected in their changing demography. In 1970 state and county mental hospitals had 413,000 beds; in 1986 and 2000 the comparable figures were 119,000 and 59,000. In 1970 there were 310 such institutions; by 2000 the number had fallen to 220. The decline in the mental hospital population was accompanied by an expansion of psychiatric facilities in general hospitals. In 1963 there were 622 short-term general hospitals with areas for inpatient psychiatric services; virtually none had specialized psychiatric units. By 1977 there were 1,056 such hospitals, and 843 had specialized inpatient psychiatric units.[13]

The decline in the number and population of mental hospitals and the corresponding expansion of general hospitals, however, is not to be construed as synonymous with deinstitutionalization. Beginning in the 1960s a series of developments facilitated the appearance of services to new populations: the growth of private and public insurance coverage for inpatient psychiatric care; an expanded definition of mental illnesses and the need for treatment; and greater public acceptance of psychiatric care. Equally if not more important in stimulating the demand for services was the extraordinarily rapid growth of clinically trained mental health personnel. In 1947 there were about 4,700 psychiatrists in the United States and in the core areas of psychiatry, clinical psychology, psychiatric social work, and psychiatric nursing, only 23,000. By 1976 the comparable figures were 11,576 and 104,061. By the end of the twentieth century the number of disciplines with clinical training had expanded even further; the total number of such individuals in these specialties exceeded 400,000. There is little doubt that the availability of services, together with the expansion of diagnostic categories in the APA's *Diagnostic and Statistical Manual of Mental Disorders* (more commonly know as *DSM-III*) in 1980 and the striking increase in the marketing of pharmaceuticals, stimulated the public demand for mental health services.[14] The result was a dramatic increase in usage by individuals, some of whom did not have a mental illness. Nor were individuals treated for psychiatric disorders in general hospitals necessarily those who would have been patients in state and county long-term mental hospitals. What actually occurred was an expansion of the mental health service system in which the relative role of public mental hospitals diminished even though their absolute role continued to endure.[15]

Nowhere were the changes in the mental health system more visible than in the aggregate data dealing with patient care episodes. In 1955 there were 1,675,352 patient care episodes. Twenty-two percent occurred in outpatient facilities, 50 percent in state mental hospitals, and the remainder in other institutions. Of 6.4 million episodes in 1977, by contrast, 72 percent occurred in outpatient facilities (of which 27 percent were in CMHCs), and only 9 percent in state mental hospitals. Despite the fall in the state hospital inpatient census, admissions continued on an upward slope. In 1955 these institutions had 559,000 patients at the end of the year. During that year there were 178,003 admissions, 126,498 releases, and 44,384 deaths. Two decades later the number of resident patients had fallen to 193,436, but admissions had nearly tripled. In other words, the number of long-stay patients fell dramatically as the number of short-stay patients increased. By the end of the 1970s state hospitals were admitting 400,000 persons annually, of whom two-thirds were readmissions.[16]

The dramatic growth of outpatient facilities did diminish the relative significance of public mental hospitals. Yet appearances were somewhat misleading. As the number of aged and chronic in public mental hospitals fell after the passage of Medicaid and Medicare, these institutions began to provide more short- and intermediate-term care and treatment for persons with severe mental illnesses. Between 1970 and 1975 the median length of stay fell from 41 to 25 days. These hospitals also still provided long-term care: state hospitals remained what three investigators termed "the place of last resort" for perhaps 100,000 individuals for whom no alternative facility was available. Thus in 1969 the mean stay of discharged patients at state hospitals was 421 days; six years later the corresponding figure was 270 days. In these same years these institutions accounted for 79 and 67 percent, respectively, of all days of inpatient psychiatric care.[17]

The increase in the number of both inpatient and outpatient care episodes at general hospitals and CMHCs did not mean that individuals previously admitted to state mental hospitals were now being treated at these facilities. On the contrary, general hospitals and CMHCs tended to be used by new groups that in the past had no access to the mental health system. Many of the changes in the mental health system, in other words, occurred because of the expansion of services and recruitment of a new clientele rather than because of the substitution of one service for another. State mental hospitals in general treated more individuals with severe and persistent mental disorders than did general hospitals or CHMCs. This patient load was reflected in both the mean and the median stays. In 1980 the mean stay at general hospitals with specialized psychiatric units was 11.6 days and the median 6.9. The comparable figures for state hospitals for that same year were 165 and 23.[18]

By the 1970s the dramatic growth of mental health facilities, the rise in usage, the decline of long-stay mental hospital populations, and the existence of a variety of federal entitlement programs seemed to herald the inauguration of a new system capable of overcoming the older deficiencies associated with long-term institutional care. Nevertheless, it was becoming increasingly evident that serious structural weaknesses in the system had the potential to vitiate the goals of providing comprehensive care and treatment for vulnerable individuals with serious and persistent mental disorders. The fact of the matter was that the mental health system lacked mechanisms that would ensure coordination or cooperation. Two decades of struggle for fundamental policy changes had led to disorganization as well as to competition between organizations and clients. By the 1970s the system included a bewildering array of institutions: state and federal institutions providing both short- and long-term care and treatment; private psychiatric hospitals; nursing homes; residential care facilities; CMHCs; outpatient and inpatient psychiatric units in general hospitals; community care programs; community residential institutions for persons with mental disorders with different designations in different states; and client-run and self-help services. The disarray and lack of any unified structure for financing or service integration only compounded the problems faced by individuals with serious disorders.

Deinstitutionalization was based on the premise that most of the patients cared for in state hospitals would do much better living in the community. Although it was clear that many patients preferred to live in the community, they faced formidable problems. Experiments in community living were by no means novel. In the late nineteenth century Massachusetts pioneered the boarding out of quiet persons with persistent mental disorders in private homes. Several other states followed suit. In 1963 twenty-three states had placed 13,292 patients with families. New York, Illinois, Michigan, and California accounted for nearly 69 percent of the total. Several thousand more had been placed in home care by the Veterans Administration. Yet family care remained a marginal activity. To oversee and supervise such programs was extremely difficult, to say nothing of community resistance to the placement of patients in their midst. Family care, therefore, never became a significant component of the mental health system.[19]

In 1954 the New York State Department of Mental Hygiene recognized that the "period of transition from hospital to community presents increased hazards for patients, leaving, as they are, a protected environment to face anew the stresses and strains of family and community living." It therefore created four aftercare clinics in New York City to deal with the more than 7,000 patients on convalescent leave.[20] At about the same time "halfway houses"—institutions designed to ease the transition of patients from hospital to community—came into existence. Such facilities grew out of the concern for discharged patients by such figures as Dr. Abraham Low (the creator of Recovery, Inc.) in the 1930s, experiences with military convalescent hospitals during World War II, and the belief that the new psychotropic drugs would facilitate the release of institutionalized patients.

Halfway houses did not necessarily have a shared set of characteristics. Some were organized under professional auspices; some had direct links with hospitals; and others were founded by laypersons. One of the most famous— Fountain House in New York City—evolved out of an informal organization of former Rockland State Hospital patients in the 1940s. In 1948 it acquired a clubhouse and acted as a support group. Later it expanded its scope by establishing a transitional employment program and acquiring residential apartments for members. By 1970 there were perhaps 170 such facilities serving about 3,000 individuals. Most had been diagnosed with schizophrenia and virtually all had been hospitalized. The average length of stay was between four and six months. In a given year, therefore, halfway houses served between 6,000 and 9,000 individuals. Despite their promise, they never became a significant component within the mental health system, if only because the system for financing mental health services made few provisions for such institutions. Most had to rely on private funding, and their financial state was always precarious. "Many mental health professionals," observed Raymond Glasscote and his associates in their study of rehabilitation for the APA in 1971, "do not have much knowledge of, interest in, or commitment to the importance of rehabilitative and supporting resources that must be available on an intermediate or long-term basis to the seriously ill people that they seek to retain in the community."[21]

The problems of the mental health system were further exacerbated by attacks upon its very legitimacy as well as a fundamental change in the nature of the population with mental disorders. During the 1960s an anti-psychiatry movement had begun to promote the concept that mental illness was a myth that served as a form of social labeling to suppress nonconformist behavior. A peculiar coalition drawn from the libertarian right and the New Left, associated with such figures as Thomas S. Szasz, R. D. Laing, Erving Goffman, and Thomas J. Scheff attempted to call into question the foundations of psychiatry. Szasz, for example, argued that the concept of mental illness was a myth and that individuals behaving in unconventional ways were being controlled by psychiatrists. Laing suggested that madness might be a rational response to an irrational world. Goffman described the ways in which a humiliating institutionalization stripped individuals of their self-identity and esteem and induced deviant responses. Scheff was an ardent exponent of "labeling" (or societal reaction) theory, which maintained that psychiatric diagnoses were merely convenient labels attached to individuals who violated conventional behavioral norms. The stigmatizing of individuals as mentally ill in turn produced disturbed behavior. Many younger street persons with mental disorders were influenced by such claims and insisted that they were being victimized because of their nonconformist behavior.[22]

Nor were attacks on psychiatric hegemony limited to external critics. By the 1960s clinical psychologists (who had come into conflict with psychiatrists in the 1950s over licensing and certification) were arguing that the medical model of mental illnesses was deficient. In insisting that they were equally, if not more, qualified to offer psychotherapy, they posed a challenge to psychiatric hegemony. In a debate with a distinguished psychiatrist, George W. Albee (a psychologist who had prepared one of the monographs for the JCMIH) rejected the illness model. He claimed that disturbed behavior reflected "the results of social-developmental learning in pathological environments." Effective interventions therefore had to be social and educational in nature; one-to-one therapeutic relationships were essentially futile. Albee's public health model, which emphasized broad interventions to restore the "emotional integrity of the family," left little room for traditional psychiatric therapies.[23]

A more subtle but equally significant critique of psychiatry came from individuals associated with the civil rights movement and members of the legal profession. In the postwar decades concern with racial, gender, and class inequality created novel definitions of rights that eventually included people with mental disorders. The new concern with patient rights was related in part to the perceived crisis of mental hospitals. If society created a system of involuntary confinement, did it not have a commensurate responsibility to provide appropriate treatment? The issue was raised by Morton Birnbaum in 1960 when he argued that involuntary confinement of a person with a mental illness without providing medical treatment was equivalent to imprisonment without substantive due process of law.[24]

Shortly thereafter there were major challenges to the procedures governing commitment, hospitalization, and treatment in both lower federal and
state courts. Advocates for persons with mental illnesses argued that commitment statutes were vague and arbitrary; that courts and legislatures should
be required to follow a "least restrictive" alternative approach to civil commitment; that all persons involuntarily committed should be provided with
due process procedures to ensure that they would not be deprived of their
liberties; and that hospitalized patients ought to retain certain basic rights,
including a right to treatment and a right to refuse treatment with medication.
Bruce Ennis, who directed the Civil Liberties and Mental Illness Litigation
Project in New York City, described the problem in stark terms. Many patients,
he wrote in 1972,

> will be physically abused, a few will be raped or killed, but most of
> them will simply be ignored, left to fend for themselves in the cheerless
> corridors and barren back wards of the massive steel and concrete ware-
> houses we—but not they—call hospitals. . . .
>
> So vast an enterprise will occasionally harbor a sadistic psychiatrist
> or a brutal attendant, condemned even by his colleagues when discov-
> ered. But that is not the central problem. The problem, rather, is the
> enterprise itself. . . . They [patients] are put away not because they are,
> in fact, dangerous, but because they are useless, unproductive, "odd,"
> or "different."[25]

Ennis's statement exaggerated the warehousing functions of public hospitals,
which, after all, did provide for the basic necessities of life for a population
whose illness created disability. Nevertheless, his words appealed to critics
of hospitals.

In the 1960s and 1970s a series of state and federal judicial decisions began
to modify long-accepted legal procedures. In *Rouse v. Cameron* the District of
Columbia Circuit Court of Appeals stipulated that mental patients committed
by criminal courts had a right to treatment. Several years later an Alabama federal district court extended the right to adequate treatment to all individuals
involuntarily confined in institutions. Dissatisfied with the state plan, the court
issued an order detailing minimum criteria for adequate treatment. Courts also
began to modify traditional commitment processes by imposing procedural
safeguards and limiting involuntary commitment to those individuals representing a danger to others or themselves. A further series of decisions defined
a right to refuse treatment.[26]

Judicial activism aroused anger and fear among psychiatrists, some of whom interpreted the changes as undermining their authority and even their legitimacy, to say nothing about disregarding the plight of individuals with severe and persistent mental disorders. Yet the consequences of reform, as Paul S. Appelbaum noted, "were much more limited than partisans on either side anticipated." Perhaps the most significant change was one of attitude. No longer could persons with mental disorders be deprived of their liberties with few procedural protections. It became axiomatic "that services must be provided in a manner that minimizes intrusions on individual rights and maximizes patients' recourse to independent review when infringements occur." Even the right to refuse treatment had a minimal impact. Judges were not disposed to veto treatment recommendations. The incidence of treatment refusal was not large, and often reflected a dislike of medication because of adverse side effects. One result of litigation was the creation of a somewhat less paternalistic relationship between psychiatrist and patient. Yet litigation did not always have a positive impact. Faced with court-mandated minimum standards of care (such as staff-patient ratios, per capita expenditures) hospital administrators often met them by discharging patients into communities ill-prepared to provide appropriate services, thus raising institutional indices without in any way remedying institutional deficiencies.[27]

Although given considerable publicity, judicial decisions in reality played at best a marginal role in shaping an increasingly complex, decentralized, and uncoordinated mental health system. The population traditionally identified as having a severe mental disorder, however, was affected in a way that was far from marginal. For over a century such individuals had received care and treatment within state mental hospitals. Indeed, the policy of deinstitutionalization—whatever its meaning—was based on the premise that the population found in mental hospitals should and could be treated in the community.

The first major wave of discharges came after 1965, and largely included individuals who had been institutionalized for relatively long periods of time or else had been admitted later in their lives. Many were relocated in chronic care facilities or else returned to the community. In its initial stage, therefore, deinstitutionalization was confined to individuals who constituted the bulk of the traditional inpatient population. This phase was not controversial and did not create difficulties, since few of these persons seemed to pose a threat to themselves or to others. Indeed, some of these individuals made a more or less successful transition from hospital to community.

Basic demographic trends in the population as a whole and changes in the mental health service system in particular created a quite different situation. At the end of World War II there was a sharp rise in the number of births that peaked in the 1960s. Between 1946 and 1960 more than fifty-nine million births were recorded. The disproportionately large size of this age cohort meant that the number of persons at risk for developing severe mental disorders was high. Morton Kramer, a distinguished epidemiologist and biostatistician, warned that large increases were to be expected between 1975 and 1990 "in numbers of persons in the high-risk age groups for the use of mental health facilities, and correctional institutions, homes for the aged and dependent and other institutions that constitute the institutional population." Moreover, younger persons tended to be highly mobile. Whereas 40 percent of the general population moved between 1975 and 1979, as many as two-thirds or more of individuals in their twenties changed residences. Like others in their age cohort, the growing numbers of young adults with a severe and persistent mental disorder also moved frequently, both within and between urban areas and in and out of rural areas.[28]

At the same time that the cohort born after 1945 was reaching its twenties and thirties, the mental health service system was undergoing fundamental changes. Until the 1960s individuals with severe and persistent mental disorders were generally cared for and treated in state mental hospitals. If admitted in their youth, they were either institutionalized for decades or discharged and then often readmitted. Under these circumstances responsibility for their care and treatment was centralized within a specific institutional context, and in general these individuals were not visible in the community at large. Some persons with severe and persistent mental illnesses did of course reside in the community. But their relatively small numbers posed few difficulties and in general their presence did not arouse public apprehension.

After 1970, however, a quite different situation prevailed. A subgroup of individuals with severe and persistent mental illnesses—composed largely of young adults—was adversely affected by the changes in the mental health service system. These individuals were rarely confined for extended periods within mental hospitals. Restless and mobile, they were the first generation of individuals with major psychiatric illnesses to reach adulthood within the community. Their disorders were not fundamentally different from those of their predecessors. Nevertheless, they behaved in very different ways. They tended to emulate the behavior of their age peers, who were often hostile toward conventions and authority. Young adults with severe disorders exhibited aggressiveness, volatility, and were noncompliant. They generally fell into the schizophrenic category, although affective disorders and borderline personalities were also present. Above all, they lacked functional and adaptive skills. A knowledgeable psychiatrist and his colleagues emphasized the dysfunctional character of these individuals. "In terms of the necessary equipment for community life—the capacity to endure stress, to work consistently toward realistic goals, to relate to other people comfortably over time, to tolerate uncertainty and conflict—these young adults are disabled in a very real and pervasive sense."[29]

Many of these young adults with severe and persistent mental disorders had high rates of alcoholism and drug abuse, which only exacerbated their volatile and noncompliant behavior. Their mobility and lack of coping skills also resulted in high rates of homelessness. Many of them traveled and lived together on the streets, thereby reinforcing each other's pathology. Urban areas in particular began to experience the presence of such individuals. But even rural states such as Vermont found that many individuals with severe and persistent disorders were made up of transients requiring treatment, welfare, and support services. An APA report on homeless persons with mental disorders emphasized the tendency of these young persons to drift.

> Apart from their desire to outrun their problems, their symptoms, and their failures, many have great difficulty achieving closeness and intimacy.
>
> They drift also in search of autonomy, as a way of denying their dependency, and out of a desire for an isolated life-style. Lack of money often makes them unwelcome, and they may be evicted by family and friends. And they drift because of a reluctance to become involved in a mental health treatment program or a supportive out-of-home environment . . . [T]hey do not want to see themselves as ill.[30]

As young adults with severe and persistent mental illnesses were becoming more prominent, the mental hospital was losing its central position and the traditional links between care and treatment were shattered. Treatment was subsumed under a decentralized medical and psychiatric service system that served a varied and diversified client population. Care, by contrast, increasingly came under the jurisdiction of a series of federal entitlement programs which presumed that income maintenance payments, access to treatment, housing, and food stamps would enable disabled persons to live in their communities. Indeed, such programs increasingly drove the process of deinstitutionalization, since the release of patients from state institutions to communities meant an implicit transfer of funding responsibilities from states to the federal government.

The combination of a decentralized psychiatric system, multiple bureaucracies with different and sometimes competing concerns, and the emergence of a young adult population with severe disorders had profound consequences. Before 1965 mental hospitals retained responsibility for this population. After 1970 many from this group tended to be pervasive but unsystematic users of psychiatric facilities. They entered and left mental hospitals in what were brief stays; they used emergency and psychiatric wards of general hospitals and other inpatient and outpatient facilities; and they could be found as well in correctional and penal institutions. Their high use of services tended to resemble a revolving door. Because of their mobility and restlessness, they moved quickly from one service to another. They proved to be noncompliant; their use of medication was sporadic and inconsistent; their refusal or inability to follow a sustained and rational treatment plan meant that the benefits gained were transient and minimal; and they often had a dual diagnosis of a serious mental disorder and substance abuse.

Such patients tended to arouse negative reactions from mental health professionals. A persistent disorder and substance abuse contradicted the medical dream of cure. The management of such young and intransigent individuals was often frustrating, creating powerful emotions of helplessness and inadequacy among professionals whose background and training had not prepared them for such a clientele. Equally significant, those who worked with these young adults received little or no peer support from their colleagues who dealt with different types of patients, and they found themselves outside the mainstream of psychiatry. "One of the highest 'costs' of the current pattern of interaction with these patients," conceded two psychiatrists,

> is the response of the caretakers themselves. As patients alternately demand and reject care, as they alternate between dependency, manipulation, withdrawal, anger, depression, and other interactive styles and emotional states, even the most tolerant and resourceful clinician is likely to experience increasing anger, bitterness, frustration, and helplessness. These responses, in turn, can lead to even more inappropriate treatment decisions, which are not in anyone's long-term interests but only serve to remove the patient, temporarily, from the responsibility of a given caretaker.[31]

Deinstitutionalization, as conceived in the postwar decades and implemented after the 1960s, assumed that individuals with severe and persistent disorders would be treated in the community; hospital stays, if necessary, would be brief. Those requiring treatment and care would be served by a series of linked and integrated aftercare institutions and programs. Such assumptions, however, hardly applied to many of the young individuals who were so visible during and after the 1970s. They had little or no experiences with prolonged institutionalization, and hence had not internalized the behavioral norms of a hospital community. To be sure, many of the norms of patienthood in institutions were objectionable, but at the very least they provided individuals with some kind of structure. Lacking such guidance, many young adults—especially those with a dual diagnosis—developed a common cultural identity quite at variance with the society in which they lived. The mobility of such individuals, the absence of a family support system, and programmatic shortcomings complicated their access to basic necessities such as adequate housing and social support networks. The dearth of many basic necessities of life further exacerbated their severe mental disorders. Ironically, at the very time that unified, coordinated, and integrated medical and social services were needed to deal with a new patient population, the policy of deinstitutionalization had created a decentralized system that often lacked any clear focus and diffused responsibility and authority.

At a superficial level the mental health initiatives of both the Kennedy and the Johnson administrations seemed to have inaugurated a new chapter insofar as the care and treatment of mentally ill persons was concerned. The increase in the number of CMHCs and the acceleration of the decline in mental hospital populations appeared to confirm the belief that the new community-oriented policy would lead in the not too distant future to the end of institutionalization. At a number of congressional hearings prominent figures expressed their gratification that the CMHC acts of 1963 and 1965 had transformed in fundamental ways the manner in which persons with severe and persistent mental disorders received care and treatment. Wilbur Cohen, acting secretary of DHEW, told a congressional committee that mental disorders had been brought "out in the open" because of the existence of community mental health services. Many persons with such disorders, he added, "can be put back to work, can be given their rightful place in society and they are not a drain on either their families or the taxpayer." Robert Finch, Cohen's successor in the Nixon administration, was equally sanguine, commenting that "one of the real successes of recent years has been the program of community mental health."[32]

Rhetoric notwithstanding, there was little or no evidence to support such optimistic claims. The decline in inpatient mental hospital populations had little to do with the slow expansion in the number of centers, most of which had only tenuous relationships with persons with serious disorders. Centers, charged APA president Donald G. Langsley in 1980, had "drifted away from their original purpose" and featured "counseling and crisis intervention for predictable problems of living." The result was a disregard of individuals with serious mental disorders. The absolute decline in the number of psychiatrists affiliated with centers was matched by an increase in psychologists and social workers. This development only vitiated still further the original mandate of centers, since psychiatrists were more likely to work with persons with severe disorders than other staff.[33]

Federal pressure could have forced CMHCs to give priority to persons with the most severe mental disorders. But the federal government lacked an administrative structure capable of overseeing the operations of local centers. State authorities might have assumed a supervisory role. Much of the legislation enacted during the halcyon decade of the 1960s, however, was based on the belief that many states were either inept or reactionary, and that a federal–local partnership could achieve far more. Under these circumstances community institutions became vulnerable to constituent pressures to provide services that dealt with personal problems and substance abuse. Individuals with severe and persistent mental disorders—a group that lacked an effective lobby capable of protecting their interests—tended to be disregarded.

Equally important, by the late 1960s federal policy began to shift markedly because of a growing perception that substance abuse (notably drugs and, to a lesser extent, alcohol) represented a major threat to the well-being of the public. Beginning in 1968 federal legislation sharply altered the role of centers by adding new services for substance abusers, children, and the elderly. Congress acted on the assumption that the CMHC acts of 1963 and 1965 had resolved most of the problems faced by persons with severe disorders and that the time had come to provide services to other groups supposedly in need of mental health services. As the mandate of centers broadened, mental health policy became less focused and more diffuse.

The political climate after 1969 added still another discordant element. In the decades after 1945 the individuals who occupied the White House tended to follow the lead of a powerful bipartisan lobby determined to expand federal biomedical research and to disseminate the benefits of modern medicine to the population as a whole. Its members had an ambitious agenda that included strong support for mental health programs. By the late 1960s, however, their power, though still formidable, had begun to ebb. The fiscal pressures associated with the Vietnam War, alleged fiscal mismanagement by NIH officials, internal differences over priorities, and the death of Representative John Fogarty and the retirement of Senator Lister Hill weakened the influence of a coalition that had made national government the major player in the health policy arena.[34] When Richard M. Nixon took office in early 1969, friction inevitably followed.

Unlike his predecessor, Nixon had an uneasy relationship with psychiatry. Psychodynamic practitioners, who still dominated the specialty, were generally associated with a liberal political ideology and committed to a variety of social programs. Moreover, some CMHCs—particularly those in larger urban areas—were associated with activist political agendas. Nixon tended to be more conservative. He wanted to consolidate many of the social programs enacted earlier rather than embarking on new experiments, except for his aborted family assistance plan. Under these circumstances it was perhaps inevitable that conflict over the proper shape of mental health policy and the role of the federal government would follow.

During his first year in office Nixon was preoccupied with the Vietnam War. Legislation providing continuing funding for construction and staffing of CHMCs passed without much controversy. In 1970, however, open conflict erupted. Stanley Yolles was forced out as director of the NIMH because of basic policy differences. Many members of the administration either opposed the social programs created during the 1960s or else believed that categorical grants were ineffective. Between 1970 and 1972 the administration worked assiduously to cut NIMH programs, most of which survived because of a friendly Congress. Differences came to a head when the administration recommended that the CMHC program be terminated forthwith. In testimony before a congressional committee, DHEW secretary Casper W. Weinberger insisted that the CMHC program had always been designed as a demonstration rather than as a permanent project. Having impounded CMHC funds, he urged an end to federal involvement and a state takeover of the administration and funding of the program. His argument that the act of 1963 was designed as a demonstration project was emphatically rejected by committee members. Their position was upheld by Judge Gerhard Gesell of the U.S. District Court for the District of Columbia, who ordered the impounded funds released. The act of 1963, he wrote, "was never viewed by Congress as a demonstration program . . . but rather [was] a national effort to redress the present wholly inadequate measures being taken to meet increasing mental health treatment needs."[35]

The conflict between the administration and Congress produced more heat than light; the claims of both protagonists rested on a shaky foundation. Defenders insisted that there was a direct relationship between CMHCs and the decline in mental hospital populations, even though data to support such an allegation were largely absent. The administration claim that the intent of the original legislation was to create a demonstration project was equally fallacious. The partisan character of the conflict inadvertently deflected attention from the plight faced by ever-growing numbers of persons with serious and persistent mental disorders living in communities and lacking integrated services that would provide food, housing, and social support networks.

While Congress was considering legislation to extend the CMHC program, continuing revelations about the Watergate scandal increasingly occupied the attention of the White House. Nixon's resignation in the summer of 1974 brought a sigh of relief from those concerned with mental health issues, if only because of the perception that his administration was an implacable enemy of a federal role in shaping and financing services. In the months preceding and following Nixon's resignation, Congress began to reassess the CMHC program because of its obvious shortcomings. The GAO, which provided studies and evaluations for Congress, noted in 1974 that a system "for the coordinated delivery of mental-health services had not been fully developed." Its report emphasized the absence of working relationships between mental hospitals and centers.[36]

In mid-1975 Congress overrode a veto by President Gerald Ford and enacted legislation that substantially altered the definition of a CMHC. The regulations governing the original act of 1963 required centers to provide five essential services. The new law mandated twelve. These included screening, follow-up care and therapy for released patients as well as specialized services for children, the elderly, and alcohol and drug abusers. A two-year grant program provided centers with temporary funding to institute these services. In 1977 and 1978 Congress extended the program's authorization for one and two years, respectively. By that time there were about 650 CMHCs, a total far below the original goal of 2,000 centers by 1980. Despite its travails, the program had survived through four presidential administrations. The 1975 legislation explicitly endorsed the goals that had been written into the law in 1963. Community mental health care, noted the preamble to the act,

> is the most effective and humane form of care for a majority of mentally ill individuals; the federally funded community mental health centers have had a major impact on the improvement of mental health by (a) fostering coordination and cooperation between agencies responsible for mental health care, which in turn has resulted in a decrease of overlapping services and more efficient utilization of available resources, (b) bringing comprehensive community mental health care to all who need care within a specific geographic area regardless of ability to pay, and (c) developing a system of care which insures continuity of care for all patients and thus our national resource to which all Americans should enjoy access.[37]

CMHCs were still officially recognized as an important component within the mental health system. Yet as limited federal resources were diverted to new centers, older ones were left in an increasingly precarious condition. More important, centers were not serving the needs of those being released in ever-growing numbers from state hospitals. The counterproductive friction between Congress and the White House prevented both sides from asking whether or not the basic human needs of a severely disabled population were being met. As deinstitutionalized patients became more visible, the need to address the issue of their care was becoming acute.

At the beginning of 1977 the GAO prepared a comprehensive report to Congress that laid bare the problems of a disorganized and uncoordinated mental health system. It endorsed deinstitutionalization, but was extraordinarily critical of the manner in which it was implemented. The most pressing need was for social support services, including suitable living arrangements, income support, vocational training, employment, protective supervision, and other services. Yet many individuals remained in hospitals because of the absence of community-based facilities and services. Even when released, "responsibility for their care and support frequently [became] diffused among several agencies and levels of government." The lack of formal links between public mental hospitals and CMHCs only exacerbated the situation. The dramatic growth of federal involvement in mental health had not produced the anticipated benefits, the report noted, if only because there was little or no coordination between the 135 federal programs administered by 11 major agencies and departments.[38]

In theory federal programs such as Medicare, Medicaid, SSI, and Title XX of the Social Security Act had great potential to facilitate community care and treatment. Nevertheless, problems with each of these programs placed impediments in the way of deinstitutionalization. Medicaid, for example, provided funding for placement of persons with mental disabilities in nursing homes and intermediate care facilities that were often unprepared to meet these individuals needs. Medicare coverage of outpatient mental health care was limited to half the cost or $250 annually, whichever was less. Such a limitation led to unnecessary hospitalization. The Social Security Act prohibited paying SSI to persons in public institutions unless their care was reimbursed under Medicaid. This provision, however, was counterproductive, for it prohibited the payment of benefits to those in group or sheltered homes, halfway houses, or hostels operated by state and local governments. There was also controversy, confusion, and disagreements between states and DHEW over what social services were eligible for federal reimbursement. Similarly, the programs administered by the Department of Housing and Urban Development (HUD) neither informed nor encouraged local housing authorities and managers to consider the needs of the mentally disabled when formulating housing plans and policies.[39]

The GAO's analysis portrayed a dysfunctional mental health system. Neither federal, state, nor local governments had developed systematic ways to finance deinstitutionalization, nor were agency roles at all levels clear or consistent. "There has been no clear, comprehensive, consistent Federal strategy for helping State and local governments to return mentally disabled persons to, or keep them in, communities."[40]

The GAO offered a series of recommendations designed to make deinstitutionalization a reality. It asked that legislative links among federal programs be created in order to ensure "that they are mutually supportive in accomplishing deinstitutionalization and that they are used to make sure that mentally disabled persons are placed in the least restrictive setting appropriate to their needs with needed support services provided most cost-effectively." GAO urged each branch of Congress to designate a committee to oversee all federal programs bearing on deinstitutionalization. All funds earmarked for mental health under the Special Health Revenue Sharing and CMHC programs should be converted into a formula grant to state mental health agencies, which would be in a better position to create an effective mental health system with an emphasis on community-based care. The GAO also insisted upon the necessity of clarifying and defining the roles and responsibilities of several federal agencies, including the Office of Management and Budget, DHEW, HUD, and the Department of Labor.[41]

The responses to the report by federal and state officials were mixed, though not unfavorable. The Office of Management and Budget was supportive of community care, but rejected a recommendation that it direct federal agencies to develop and implement an interdepartmental objective for accomplishing deinstitutionalization. DHEW officials felt that states had to take the lead in addressing deinstitutionalization. HUD and Labor indicated their willingness to work with DHEW, and the Department of Justice reported that it was taking an active role in an effort to establish as a constitutional principle the right to receive treatment in a least restrictive setting. The National Association of State Mental Health Program Directors, by contrast, agreed that the report represented the views of most states, but reiterated its long-standing position that federal programs should not bypass state and local governments. It also called for simplification in the flow of federal funds and criticized the legislative changes made in the CMHC program in 1975 that mandated new services but failed to provide adequate funding.[42]

Since 1945 mental health advocates had struggled to replace an institutional with a community-based policy. In some respects their hostility toward mental hospitals was understandable, even though they failed for the most part to understand the significance of the caring functions or the character of patient populations of these institutions. Moreover, activists were never fully cognizant of the difficulties of implementing a community policy, nor were they aware of the implications of expanding diagnostic categories that in effect began the process of pathologizing many behaviors previously defined as bad habits or vices.

Beginning with the passage of the CMHC Act of 1963 and the Medicare and Medicaid legislation two years later, the federal government had assumed a leading role in the mental health arena. To be sure, the federal presence was in part a result of a serendipitous process. Medicaid and other entitlement programs, which turned out to provide substantial resources for persons with mental disorders, had not been designed for this purpose. Whatever the programs' origins, however, these entities became a vital component of the mental health system. Yet the absence of program coordination and support services for persons with severe disorders vitiated their importance. Similarly, CMHCs failed to meet the expectations of those who had fought for their creation. They provided occupational opportunities for nonmedical practitioners as well as novel services for new clients who believed that mental health therapies could alleviate many everyday problems in living, but for the most part ignored individuals with the greatest disabilities and most in need of services. The basic premise that it was possible and useful to provide most treatment in community settings was not unsound if in fact reasonable systems of community care had been developed. But few communities had the foresight or commitment to finance and provide such services. Patients were left to find their way among an uncoordinated array of programs, providers, and services that happened to be available. In many cases patients who remained sick and disabled had to fend on their own, often with unfortunate consequences. As the GAO report implied, the policies adopted with hope and enthusiasm during the previous two decades had contributed to the decline in long-stay patients in state mental hospitals, but had failed to put in place alternatives. The plight faced by individuals with severe and persistent mental disorders would soon be thrust to the fore by the inauguration of a new president whose wife was committed to changing the mental health system.

Chapter 3

A Presidential Initiative

The election of Jimmy Carter in 1976 augured well for those seeking to change a dysfunctional mental health system. One of his first acts after taking office was to create a presidential commission to recommend a more effective national mental health policy. Although several previous commissions had dealt with health-related issues, none had focused on the mental health system. The hope was that a group endowed with a presidential blessing could come up with a plan to strengthen a fragmented system responsible for the care and treatment of large numbers of individuals whose severe disorders had rendered them dependent upon others for their very survival.

The establishment of a presidential commission was not a novel act. From the very beginning of the federal government, presidents had employed such commissions when answers to difficult problems were obscure, when constituent demands became extreme, or when it was deemed important to provide a breathing period in order to develop ways of dealing with pressing issues. Commissions also played an important symbolic role by indicating presidential awareness and concern. To be sure, their achievements were mixed. Yet their work led to important legislative initiatives, the implementation of significant administrative changes, and sometimes altered the social and political environment. During the 1960s and early 1970s, for example, presidential commissions focused attention on assassinations, race relations, urban riots, violence, campus unrest, obscenity and pornography, and drug abuse.[1]

Carter's interest in mental illnesses and retardation had long-standing roots. Two first cousins had mental disorders and another was retarded, and they had been institutionalized for much of their lives. At the time that Carter became governor of Georgia, the state's mental health system, like those in many southern states, left much to be desired. One of his earliest acts was to appoint a Commission to Improve Services to the Mentally and Emotionally Retarded. His wife, Rosalynn, decided to make mental health reform her personal priority and persuaded her husband to appoint her to the commission. During Carter's term as governor, the number of hospitalized patients declined about 30 percent and a large number of CMHCs were established. As early as 1974 Rosalynn Carter had already decided that if her husband was successful in his quest to be elected president, she would continue to focus on mental health reform. Her hope was that the seemingly beneficial results of deinstitutionalization and creation of CMHCs in Georgia could be replicated on the national level.[2]

Mental health enjoyed at best a subordinate position on Carter's presidential agenda. His wife, however, was an admirer of Eleanor Roosevelt, and was determined to take an active role as First Lady. She was concerned generally with groups that had been underserved by government, and individuals with mental illnesses and emotional problems in particular. Like her husband, she was preoccupied as well with human and women's rights, and was a strong supporter of the Equal Rights Amendment. Her close relationship with her husband and her strong personality and work ethic ensured that she would play a significant political role. Nevertheless, her knowledge of the mental health system was relatively limited. She had accepted the prevailing assumption that CMHCs could offer more effective treatments of persons with serious mental disorders than could traditional mental hospitals, a belief based largely on ideology rather than empirical evidence.[3]

Through Peter Bourne, a psychiatrist who served as Carter's advisor on mental health and drug abuse policy, Rosalynn Carter was introduced to Thomas E. Bryant and indicted a desire to become involved in an effort to transform mental health policy in the event her husband won the election. Bryant had received both a medical and a law degree from Emory University, but was disinterested in pursuing a career in either profession. While in law school he had been employed at an Atlanta community action agency. Moving to Washington toward the close of the Johnson administration, he headed the Health Affairs Office of the Office of Economic Opportunity. Bryant had planned to return to Atlanta after the election of 1968, but was persuaded to remain in that position for a year by Donald Rumsfeld, then head of that agency in the early years of the Nixon administration. In 1971 Bryant became president of the Drug Abuse Council, an organization that received most of its support from the Ford Foundation.[4]

Bryant recognized that his organization lacked the resources necessary to launch a national effort to transform mental health policy. Following Carter's election, he sought the counsel of John W. Gardner. Secretary of DHEW in the Johnson administration, Gardner played an important role in implementing many of the major legislative initiatives associated with Johnson's Great Society program, and subsequently founded the group Common Cause. He suggested that the incoming president create a national commission, an action that would not cost a significant amount of money. Another possibility was to conduct a study of the mental health system under the auspices of the Institute of Medicine of the National Academy of Sciences. After some discussion a decision was made that it would be best to create a presidential commission. Because it would have taken a year or more to get congressional authorization, Carter decided to issue an executive order creating the commission. In retrospect, Bryant believed that it would have been wiser to seek congressional approval, which might have laid the foundations for a national consensus.[5]

On February 17, 1977, Carter issued an executive order creating the President's Commission on Mental Health (PCMH). The very title suggested a fundamental shift in emphasis. Nearly two decades earlier the JCMIH had focused its attention largely on the problems faced by individuals with serious and persistent mental disorders, many of whom were institutionalized. The decision in 1977 to use the term *mental health* rather than *mental illness* in the title suggested a policy shift, even though there was virtually no recognition of its implications. The concept of mental health was based on a public health model that emphasized the role of environment, social services, and prevention, and included far more than severe and persistent mental disorders.

Mental health, of course, was a somewhat amorphous concept capable of being defined in a multitude of ways. Its imprecision and vague boundaries made it possible for a variety of advocates and organizations to claim that their concerns fell under its rubric. Severe and persistent mental illness, by contrast, was a much narrower designation; the population included within this category was more clearly identifiable. The concept of mental health also blurred important distinctions. It suggested that mental health priorities had to take into account a variety of groups and problems. Under these circumstances persons with severe and persistent mental illnesses, who previously had been at the center of public policy, were forced to compete, often unsuccessfully, with other groups that now defined their needs in terms of mental health.

Composed of twenty members, the commission was authorized to hold public hearings and conduct studies dealing with the "mentally ill, emotionally disturbed, and mentally retarded." Its members had a broad rather than a narrow mandate, and they were asked to focus on a variety of issues. Were the mentally ill, emotionally disturbed, and mentally retarded being served or underserved? What were the projected needs for dealing with emotional stress during the next twenty-five years? What was the proper role of the federal government? How could a "unified approach to all mental health and people-helping services" be developed? What kind of research was needed? How could the educational system, volunteer agencies, and other institutions minimize "emotional disturbance"? How much would it cost to change the system and how might expenditures be allocated among the three levels of government? The commission's recommendations were to be presented in a final report to the president.[6]

Having authorized the creation of the commission, Carter decided to appoint his wife as chairperson. On the day of the announcement, a large reception was planned to which all national mental health organizations had been invited. Two hours prior to the event, however, Attorney General Griffin Bell phoned the White House and informed the president that he could not name his wife as chairperson because it might have an influence on public policy. Given this situation, Carter decided that Bryant—who was originally selected as the executive director—would become chair and his wife the honorary chairperson.[7]

The selection of Bryant proved fortunate. His personal qualities endeared him to both his colleagues and his commissioners. "He had an extraordinary ability to build a consensus," recalled Paul Danaceau. Bryant, he added, was "a very genuine kind of person . . . a terrific boss . . . [and] an enormously bright guy."[8] Danaceau's observations were not usual. Although the twenty commissioners did not always agree with one another, their deliberations were never hostile or divisive, largely because of Bryant's diplomatic traits and his ability to forge a consensus.

The first task was to select twenty individuals to serve as commissioners. Gardner felt that it would be unwise for either Rosalynn Carter or Bryant to undertake this delicate task. The latter then appointed an ad hoc screening committee chaired by Gardner. Its members included Eleanor Holmes Norton (New York City Human Rights commissioner), Margaret Mahoney (vice president of the Robert Wood Johnson Foundation), Brian O'Connell (executive director of the Mental Health Association), and two well-known psychiatrists—Joseph T. English of St. Vincent's Hospital in New York City and Daniel X. Freedman, chair of the Department of Psychiatry at the University of Chicago.[9]

The selection process proved to be anything but simple. The makeup of the commission, after all, would in many ways shape both the character of its deliberations and the nature of the final recommendations. Nor did the selection process occur in a social or political vacuum. A variety of constituencies—professional, ethnic, racial, and gender—wanted their interests to be represented. Similarly, members of Congress wanted to ensure that at least one individual from their state be appointed. Bryant responded tactfully to communications from members of Congress, noting that each of the various task panels (which were in the process of being appointed) included one of their constituents.[10]

Ultimately more than a thousand names were submitted to the ad hoc committee by individuals as well as by private and public organizations, of which forty-four were sent to the White House. Because Gardner and Bryant did not want psychiatrists to dominate the commission, they developed some general guidelines to guide the deliberations of the ad hoc committee and to ensure that individuals from diverse backgrounds and groups be selected.[11]

The composition of the commission reflected in many ways the group consciousness that had become so pervasive by the 1970s. The twenty commissioners came from diverse backgrounds, and their interests revolved around the mental health of minorities and underserved groups rather than the specific needs of persons with severe and persistent mental illnesses. In this respect it was unlike the JCMIH or the panel on mental retardation, both of which played important roles during the Kennedy administration. In the 1950s and early 1960s it was possible for individuals to drive policy. Thus Robert H. Felix and Eunice Shriver played key roles in the passage of the act of 1963 that provided federal funds for the construction of facilities designed to provide services to individuals with severe mental disorders and developmental disabilities. The PCMH, by contrast, was created in a different environment. By the 1970s a wide array of constituencies, professional groups, and congressional figures had varying agendas. The work of the commission, therefore, reflected the politics of ethnic, gender, and racial diversity.

In terms of gender, the commission had twelve men and eight women. Three commissioners were African American, two were Hispanic, and one was a Native American. The occupational and professional backgrounds of the members varied in the extreme. A majority were involved with mental health, although their interests were dissimilar. Priscilla Allen, a former patient, had been deeply involved in mental health policy in California, and served as an advocate for persons with mental disorders. Alan Beigel, director of the Arizona Mental Health Center, was active in policy issues and had taught at various institutions and written numerous articles. George Tarjan had spent most of his career at UCLA; he had served on Kennedy's panel on mental retardation and his interdisciplinary research dealing with the treatment of individuals with developmental disabilities—notably children and adolescents—gave him a national reputation. Mildred Mitchell-Bateman, commissioner of the West Virginia Department of Mental Health and a well-known African American psychiatrist, was concerned with underserved populations. Julius B. Richmond was a noted pediatrician and child psychiatrist at Harvard and a key figure in founding Head Start and creating Neighborhood Health Centers. Shortly after joining the commission he was appointed assistant secretary of health in DHEW. Beverly Long, an activist in mental health affairs in Georgia, had a close relationship with the Carters. Florence Mahoney, an advocate for the needs of the aged and a major figure in promoting biomedical research, had also been co-chair of the National Committee Against Mental Illness for nearly three decades. Martha Mitchell, a psychiatric nursing administrator at Yale, was concerned with the role of nursing in mental health delivery care.

The remaining members of the PCMH came from different occupational and professional backgrounds. Jose Cabranes, an attorney, served as general counsel and director of government relations at Yale and was a specialist in the regulation of hospital costs. John Conger, a child development expert at the University of Colorado School of Medicine, had written extensively on child and adolescent health problems. Thomas Conlan, a trial lawyer, was a member of Alcoholics Anonymous and an activist in problems of alcoholism. Virginia Dayton, chairperson of the board of directors of the Bach Institute in Minneapolis, was a specialist in family systems theory and care systems. LaDonna Harris, a member of the Comanche tribe, was recognized as a crusader for human rights and for Native Americans, and served on numerous advocacy boards. Ruth B. Love, an African American educator concerned with disadvantaged and minority youth, was superintendent of schools in Oakland, California. Harold Richman, a social welfare policy expert and dean at the University of Chicago School of Social Service Administration, had been a White House Fellow and special assistant to the secretary of labor from 1965 to 1967. Reymundo Rodriguez, health educator and urban planner at the Hogg Foundation for Mental Health at the University of Texas at Austin, was involved in a variety of educational, civic, and philanthropic activities. Franklin E. Vilas, a New York City Episcopalian minister, was known for his work in pastoral counseling. Glenn Watts, president of the Communication Workers of America, was also active in Democratic Party politics and had been an early supporter of Jimmy Carter.

Charles V. Willie, a sociologist and professor at the Harvard Graduate School of Education, had written extensively on a range of social problems.[12]

With only a few exceptions the individuals appointed to the PCMH had had little direct contact with a mental health system that lacked coherence, and their knowledge of severe and persistent mental disorders was at best rudimentary. Although it would have been inappropriate for the PCMH to have been dominated by members of the psychiatric establishment, their absence suggests that the commissioners chosen would be less prone to question claims that rested on ideology rather than on empirical data. A number of commissioners believed that poverty, racism, lack of access to services, and discrimination constituted mental health problems, and that a broad agenda of social change was required.

The composition of the PCMH created some concern within the APA. Prior to the public announcement of the commission members, Bryant met with the association's legislative representatives. He pointed out that about a quarter of the members were mental health professionals (psychiatry, psychology, psychiatric social work). "I think it reflects the make up of American society." Psychiatry, he added, was fortunate in having three members from its ranks on the commission, a statement that many of the psychiatrists present found "less than reassuring."[13]

The diversity of the commission's composition ensured that its deliberations would be wide ranging, if not diffuse. At the initial briefing in March 1977, members summarized their priorities. Pointing to his background in pediatrics and child psychiatry, for example, Julius Richmond noted that "prevention, early detection, and early remediation of emotional problems would reduce the burdens both in human terms and in dollars." Schools, Ruth Love insisted, had to provide "a more humane climate . . . to help foster mental health." Some members expressed the belief that economic cycles, war, racism, sexism, elitism, poverty, stigmatization, alcoholism, and an inadequate health system contributed to the prevalence of mental disorders. Others emphasized the fragmentation within the mental health community, the need to develop new programs and services, the problems faced by rural populations, and the persistence of stigmatization. Toward the close of the meeting Bryant pointed out that the commission could not "remedy all social and economic problems" and emphasized "the need for specific recommendations with a specific focus." A combination of pragmatism and idealism was required, and he suggested that presidential commissions that focused on specific problems and developed appropriate recommendations had a much better chance of success.[14]

The appointment of commissioners and the adoption of an agenda were only a beginning. The President's executive order establishing the PCMH offered at best a general outline rather than a specific agenda. The commission had to find sources of financing, hire a staff, and determine the manner in which it would go about its work. Conflicting bureaucratic forces added another level of complexity. White House staff members were not always receptive to mental health initiatives, because they felt that such issues might detract from more important elements of the president's agenda. The fact that Rosalynn Carter was determined to ensure the commission's success, however, served to mitigate conflict, because she had the full support of her husband.

At the outset Joseph Califano, secretary of DHEW, wanted the commission placed under his jurisdiction, but Bryant managed to maintain its independence. "It is of critical importance," he wrote to Margaret McKenna (an assistant White House counsel) " . . . to have a broad base for support and involvement. It is equally important, in my view, for this study to be demonstrably independent of the agencies which will inevitably be the target or focus of much of our analysis and final recommendations." Bryant did agree, however, to appoint a staff member to serve as a liaison between the commission and a DHEW Advisory Committee on National Health Insurance Issues.[15]

Having ensured the commission's independence, Bryant was faced with a multitude of tasks. The ad hoc character of the commission and absence of a formal congressional appropriation remained a perennial problem throughout its existence. Funding came from several sources. At the outset Bryant decided that he would not draw any salary, but would continue in his position as president of the Drug Abuse Council. Carter provided $100,000 from his discretionary account. Following a White House directive, Califano reluctantly provided additional money for operations and staff. Bryant also secured permission to tap foundation and private sources of funding. His staff consisted of twenty-four individuals, eight of whom were from DHEW, which paid their salary, and sixteen full-time employees. Bryant was cognizant of the fact that the commission would have to direct its work not only to a professional audience but to a broad public and political constituency as well. To edit and remove the professional and technical jargon from its reports, he hired Paul Danaceau, who had both a journalism and a political background. Danaceau's role was to make sure that all of the PCMH's reports were written in a clear and literate manner and were accessible to a broad public.[16]

The basic work that would presumably serve as the foundation for the final report was to be done by a series of task panels that drew upon the expertise of individuals from a variety of backgrounds and disciplines. Such panels enhanced the PCMH's legitimacy. Using private foundation funding, Bryant hired two deputy directors, both of whom were psychiatrists. Beatrix (Betty) Hamburg, from Stanford University's School of Medicine, oversaw the task panels dealing with support and minority groups. Gary Tischler, from Yale University, oversaw the research and finance panels. Steven Sharfstein, then at the NIMH, also worked with the commission. All helped find appropriate individuals to serve on the task panels and subsequently worked with them. On occasion Bryant had to mediate differences among the staff. Generally speaking, however, the PCMH functioned efficiently.[17]

The task panels were both thematic and constituency driven. At the outset there was a firm conviction that the PCMH had to have a strong public representation in addition to a professional presence. Public concerns in mental health tended to be much broader than those of professionals. "One needed to reconcile or at least provide a voice for the diverse groups speaking to or complaining about issues relating to a broadly defined view of what constituted a reasonable definition of [the] mental health of the nation," recalled Tischler. "It was not to be merely a clinical Weltanschauung." The "public," after all, was composed of diverse groups, each with a different outlook. The structure of the commission, therefore, reflected both political and professional interests.[18]

Each task panel had as many as fifteen members, one of whom acted as the coordinator, with a staff member assigned for research and support. Ultimately nearly two dozen task panels were formed, with some having several subpanels. They were organized thematically, and covered subjects such as the nature and scope of mental health problems, community support systems, service delivery, personnel, cost and financing, the mental health of families, special populations (minorities, women, physically handicapped), the elderly, Vietnam veterans, rural mental health, legal and ethical issues, research, prevention, the role of the media in promoting mental health, arts in therapy, and states' mental health issues.

More than 250 individuals representing the professions, academia, and the public—many of whom had made important contributions—served on these panels. Each panel was charged with the task of preparing a detailed report justifying its recommendations and providing "substantiation as to rationale, data base, existing and pending legislation, affected agencies, implementing agencies, projected costs, and other matters." The work of the panels was designed to serve as the basis of the commission's final report.[19]

Bryant was cognizant that Congress would play a key role in implementing the commission's recommendations. At the outset he wrote to many members of Congress asking them to identify issues they considered important. The responses varied in the extreme. A number of concerns were raised, including financing, research, rehabilitation, the lack of facilities in rural areas, the breakup of the family unit, and the survival of CMHCs. It was also clear that many legislators shared an expansive concept of mental health that transcended the problems associated with serious and persistent mental illnesses. Subsumed under the rubric of mental health were the retarded, children, the aged, epileptics, alcoholics, and individuals with developmental disabilities.[20]

In the months following its establishment, the commission met periodically to lay out an agenda. The specific purpose of its first official working meeting on April 19, 1977, was to define the scope of its deliberations, create the task panels, and review the development of the CMHC program.[21] The meeting began with a paper written by Betty Hamburg seeking to distinguish between those with severe mental illness and those less severely ill, and the relationships between mental hospitals and community programs. Outside some desultory discussions dealing with definitions of mental health and mental illness, prevention, and the relationship of the commissioners to the task panels, the group tended to focus on the needs of persons with serious and persistent mental illnesses and the role of CMHCs at this meeting.

Priscilla Allen, who had expressed her reservations about the problems of community care in California several years earlier,[22] observed that Hamburg's conceptualization may have been "logically correct," but did "not correspond with what actually happens in reality." Individuals with schizophrenia were rarely treated by psychiatrists, many of whom believed that the psychoses were not particularly amenable to psychiatric treatment. CMHCs, moreover, treated the "unhappy healthy." What was required was an integrated system that linked the psychiatrist with a range of services such as housing, vocational rehabilitation, and nutritional advice. Allen suggested that it would be worthwhile to think in terms of a different sort of profession "that could link the psychiatrist, whose services the psychotic persons does need at times, with . . . housing, vocational rehabilitation, [and] nutritional advice." At this juncture Tischler provided an analysis of the CMHC program since its inception, the problems posed by federal-state-community relationships, and the absence of any linkages with state hospitals. The discussions suggested that the problems of individuals with severe and persistent mental disorders had the potential to take center stage. But it was also clear that other concerns could steer the commission in quite different directions.[23]

Aware of the need to develop a broad base of support, the commission held four public hearings in different parts of the country, each lasting a day. Such hearings were designed to enlist the assistance of professional and paraprofessional groups, consumers, volunteers, and citizens, in addition to providing valuable information. Bryant also arranged press briefings in order to build public interest in the PCMH's work. The goal was to have a preliminary report ready by September 1977 and a final report by the following April.[24]

The first two hearings took place in Philadelphia and Nashville in late May, and were followed by meetings in San Francisco and Tucson a month later. Rosalynn Carter and Bryant were present at all the meetings, and they were usually joined by more than half the commissioners. Because the format permitted a variety of organizations and individuals to testify, the meetings had no particular focus. At each more than three dozen individuals testified, and others presented written communications. Some of the testimony revolved around the needs of persons with serious mental illnesses. But the overwhelming majority of the witnesses were preoccupied with concerns that were far removed from serious mental disorders.[25]

At the Philadelphia meeting, Dr. Leon Soffer, deputy health commissioner of the city's Office of Mental Health and Mental Retardation, emphasized the need for adequate aftercare services for persons with chronic mental disabilities residing in the community. Existing community care systems, he noted, were incapable of providing services because of the inability to shift funds from institutions. Average per capita expenditure at the latter was $23,000; the comparable figure for nearly 65,000 clients in the city was $390. Soffer, however, did not distinguish between those persons who were institutionalized with serious disorders and those persons in the community, most of whom did not have a serious mental illness. What was required, he insisted, was single-stream funding that would permit the transfer of resources from institutions to the community on the basis of the clients being served. Existing services (including housing) had to be integrated if individuals were to receive appropriate care. Soffer's concerns were echoed by others. But the majority of presenters, by contrast, were preoccupied with different issues. Some spoke on behalf of the mental health needs of children, women, the aged, the mentally retarded, the Hispanic community, and the Pacific Asian community. Others emphasized the need for

prevention, research, manpower and training, advocacy, and counseling services. Still others spoke about mental health on the job, renewal of the CMHC
legislation, alcoholism, and legal and ethical issues. One individual representing the Alliance for the Liberation of Mental Patients insisted that institutional
psychiatry was simply a means of social control.[26]

The concerns of those who testified at the three subsequent hearings were
similar to those expressed in Philadelphia, with the differences reflecting dissimilar regional interests. In Nashville, for example, the initial presenter emphasized the inadequacies of the service delivery system and its impact on
rural Americans with mental and emotional difficulties, and the failure of those
in policymaking positions to recognize them. In Tucson the mental health of
Native Americans, Mexican Americans, and Spanish-speaking migrants occupied center stage. In San Francisco Kenja Murase, the principal investigator
of the Pacific/Asian Coalition (an NIMH-funded national organization), spoke
about the historic discrimination faced by his varied constituency and the fact
that many were immigrants who were at high risk for mental health problems.
"May I point out to you," he told the commission in sharp language, "that the
fact of our continued exclusion from full participation in the larger society, as
symbolized by our exclusion from this Commission, more than any other factor, adversely affects the state of our mental health."[27]

Admittedly, many of the presentations emphasized shared problems. But
the list of concerns was extraordinarily broad: the mental health problems of
migrants, ethnic minorities, children, the elderly; substance abuse; teenage
pregnancy; sex offenders; the role of schools; alternatives to institutionalization; the need for research; manpower issues; patient rights; contradictory federal, state, and local laws; funding issues; the problems faced by individuals
with chronic mental illnesses; the mental health needs of gay men and lesbi-
ans; and the difficulties of CMHCs, to cite only a few. There was a recognition
that fragmentation of services and multiple funding sources constituted major
problems. The testimony of Frank Lanterman was suggestive. A member of the
California legislature, Lanterman had played an important policy role since the
1950s in sponsoring legislation designed to shift mental health services from
state hospitals to the community and to transform a commitment process that
fostered "neglect and preventive detention." Yet the results had been counterproductive, because "the dollar has not followed the patient." He urged the
commission to consider recommending block grants to states and counties for
community mental health programs, and opposed legislation that imposed the
same regulations for all fifty states in an effort to make them "all fit into the

same hat." Lanterman's analysis, however cogent, was not typical. Most of the individuals who appeared tended to offer remedies that mirrored their own interests and affiliations.[28]

Rosalynn Carter's presence at all of the public hearings enhanced the importance of the PCMH. Her devotion to the cause, however, went further. She attended virtually all of the commission's private meetings, and spoke and wrote about the need for action. She had her own independent agenda, in which mental health reform played a central role. Although she admired Eleanor Roosevelt, her position was somewhat different. Both women had an abiding interest in the poor and downtrodden. But Eleanor Roosevelt was not a part of her husband's administration; her activities reflected her own individual concerns. Rosalynn Carter, by contrast, complemented her husband's agenda, and her presence gave the PCMH a legitimacy it might otherwise not have had.[29]

The commission's members were enthusiastic about the hearings. They believed the hearings served important functions by providing useful data and valuable perspectives, focusing attention on mental health problems, and drawing in a large and diverse constituency to the deliberative process. Yet the varied nature of the testimony presented by individuals and organizations, each representing different interests, did not result in a clear agenda to guide the PCMH's work. There was a consensus that the fragmentation within the mental health system and the absence of links between clients and services were serious problems. But there was little effort to distinguish between the needs of various groups; instead, the discussion centered on underserved groups without in any way prioritizing them. Privately, some commissioners talked about the mental health needs of children and adolescents; ethnic, racial, and geographic minorities; the importance of better management; a greater emphasis on prevention; the lack of services in jails and correctional facilities; and the stress and mental disorders caused by unemployment, inadequate education, poor housing, racism, sexism, and elitism. All the commissioners implicitly accepted the claim that effective therapeutic advances and preventive interventions existed, and that new systems of financing and administration could facilitate their deployment. Finally, they agreed that deinstitutionalization was the preferred policy, and that CMHCs were "the most beneficial and accessible of present service delivery systems."[30]

One issue that proved particularly troublesome was the question of boundaries. How could mental problems that were medical in origin be distinguished from those that were societal? Willie, for example, believed that the PCMH could not avoid dealing with unemployment, inadequate education, poor housing, racism, and sexism, all of which produced stress and served as barriers to effective services. Children, the elderly, racial and ethnic minorities, and recent immigrants were high-risk populations "because of their exposure to stress-producing circumstances and the absence of institutional support." Beigel was supportive of this point of view and believed that a more expansive concept of mental health would result in greater public awareness of the need to examine their lives and thus recognize stress-producing behaviors. Allen, by contrast, saw real dangers in broadening mental health concepts; the result might result in an increase in stigmatization. She argued that the survival of individuals with severe disorders ought to take priority, and she feared that the commission's deliberative sessions and emphasis on prevention and early detection would deflect attention from dealing with that population's pressing needs.[31]

By this time concern with the problems associated with deinstitutionalization was mounting. The previous year an action paper from the New York district branch of the APA proposed that the APA place a high priority on dealing with patients with chronic mental illnesses. John A. Talbott, one of its sponsors and a figure known for his concern for patients with long-term mental illnesses, then chaired a committee to arrange for a conference. On June 8, 1977, the PCMH agreed to act with the APA as a co-sponsor. The conference was held in early January 1978; its participants included Steven S. Sharfstein (director of the Division of Mental Health Service Programs at the NIMH), who assisted in providing PCMH staff with data regarding federal mental health programs.[32]

The policy recommendations that emerged from the deliberations of the Ad Hoc Committee on the Chronic Mental Patient were notable for their relative simplicity and focus on patients with chronic mental disorders. "The assurance of care, treatment, and rehabilitation of the chronically mentally ill," the conference concluded, "is a national public health responsibility. . . . [and] every level of government bears some responsibility to assure adequate services to this population." Indeed, the final report of the PCMH dealing with the problems posed by chronic mental illnesses was indebted to the work of this committee.[33]

In July and August 1977 the commission met to receive briefings on the work of the various task panels. Because there were twenty such panels and subpanels, the commissioners did not meet as a group, but rather were assigned to individual panels on the basis of their expressed interests.[34] At these meetings they were urged to support a large number of initiatives. George Albee, a psychologist who had also been involved with the JCMIH, for example, reported on the work of the Task Panel on Prevention. He argued that no disorder had ever been brought under control by attempts to treat afflicted individuals. Only a public health strategy designed "to discover the causes and then take steps to remove the causes, or alternatively to build up resistance in individuals" could succeed. Stress, for example, played an important etiological role; hence a stress-reduction strategy could decrease the incidence of mental disorders. Virtually nothing was being done in the area of primary prevention despite the fact that such activities were far less costly than treatment. The group accepted Albee's assertion that knowledge about the prevention of mental disorders had reached a stage that made it feasible to develop specific programs, even though this claim rested largely on an ideological rather than on an empirical foundation. The recommendation that a federal office of prevention be established drew strong support, although the precise bureaucratic location of such an office was left for future consideration.[35]

The diverse nature of the task panel reports made it difficult for commissioners, particularly some of the lay members, to assimilate the many claims and recommendations. "Most of the papers we have received," observed Cabranes, "tend to be rather discursive and . . . even in those papers where there is a quite clearly delineated conclusion, or recommendations section, the recommendations tend to be rather hortatory in nature. . . . I think generally . . . we have to move from the big picture to narrow, boring, pedestrian, but presumably significant recommendations."[36] The reporter who covered the July meeting for the APA wrote that the commission was somewhat impaired by the "inexperience" of members. Its members seemed to ignore strictly psychiatric issues such as treatment, and adopted instead a working definition of mental health that included "all sorts of social and even economic dysfunction."[37] In this respect the PCMH reflected the antiprofessional ethos prominent in the 1960s and 1970s.

The varied makeup and competing interests of the commissioners and task panel members made it difficult to come to any clear and definitive recommendations. Bryant, who had to deliver a preliminary report to President Carter in mid-September, noted that the drafting of such a document was "a real hassle . . . with staff versus Commission and Commissioners disagreeing among themselves and with me."[38] He had to take into account not only the deliberations that accompanied the task panel briefings but the views of the individual commissioners. For Beverly Long the most important priority was to develop an awareness of the fact that a very large proportion of health problems were "mental-emotional."

Too often health was defined in physical terms and mental health was equated with insanity. LaDonna Harris, by contrast, was preoccupied with the problems faced by Native Americans. Thomas Conlan emphasized the role of social stress and family disintegration as a source of mental health problems. He favored an expansive interpretation of mental health that transcended a medical foundation, and insisted that mental health problems could not be alleviated without commensurate attention to social and economic problems.[39]

By the beginning of September Bryant had completed a preliminary report, which he and Rosalynn Carter delivered to and discussed with President Carter on the morning of September 15. Bryant reported that the president "was very pleased and enthusiastic about the Report and our work." That meeting was followed by a public briefing by Rosalynn Carter at the Washington Press Club. Mental health, she insisted, was much more than the absence of mental illness. Everyone "will be affected by a depression, marital problems, delinquent children, drug and alcohol related stress, the inability to deal with a death or a serious accident or an illness, or simply low esteem." Services, she added, should be provided to all troubled individuals and without the stigmatization that traditionally attached to mental health care. The media had an important role to play by providing accurate information and helping to diminish an obsolete stigmatization that posed so many barriers.[40]

The preliminary report noted that mental health problems were not limited merely to those with mental illnesses and psychiatric disorders, but also included individuals who suffered the effects of a variety of societal ills such as poverty and discrimination based on race, sex, class, age, and mental and physical handicaps. As much as 15 percent of the population (or 20 to 32 million people) required some form of mental health care, to say nothing about the 6 million who were mentally retarded. Perhaps 15 percent of school-aged children needed help for psychological disorders. The elderly in particular had a higher incidence of mental health problems, and the social and economic problems faced by minorities increased their vulnerability to psychological and emotional distress.[41]

During the previous two decades, the report continued, remarkable strides had been made in the mental health field. Basic research had contributed to broader and more effective psychological and pharmacological treatments. There had been a shift toward community-based care, symbolized by the CMHC program, and other federal initiatives—including Medicare, Medicaid, SSDI, and SSI—had made it possible to provide more care in local communities. The civil rights and consumer movements, moreover, had accelerated the discharge of patients from state hospitals. But the movement toward community care and treatment of persons with mental illnesses, no matter how beneficial, was not without its own unique problems.[42]

Four general problem areas required attention. The first was the delivery of community-based mental health services. The deficiencies in coordinating the many programs that had an impact on individuals with mental health and emotional problems mandated federal action. The report recommended the creation of an interagency group within the federal government to coordinate these programs; the encouragement of states and localities to develop more group care housing; adequate funding for CMHCs; and manpower training programs for professionals and minority mental health personnel to work in community programs. The second problem area was financing. For this the report supported the inclusion of mental health benefits in public and private insurance plans and studies that assessed the costs of providing services in different settings and organizations. The third problem area was the need to expand the knowledge base, so it urged higher levels of funding for a number of federal agencies and the NIH. Finally, the report proposed that greater efforts be made to identify strategies that would help to prevent mental disorder and disability.[43]

Even before the preliminary report was issued, the commission's work had begun to receive criticism. In early August the National Coalition of Hispanic Mental Health and Human Services Organizations sponsored a conference attended by CMHC directors and organizations representing ethnic minorities. Bryant agreed to attend and answer questions. According to some participants, the PCMH was flawed in its composition as well as in the manner in which it addressed ethnic concerns. It also had not "adequately considered the relationship between unemployment, education, economic class divisions, and other societal factors as causes of mental illness." Rufus King, head of the Los Angeles Fanon Research and Development Center, expressed unease about what would happen after the commission completed its work. Rodolpho B. Sanchez, national director of the coalition, was even more critical. "Nothing is going to be done for us. We've got to seek other avenues."[44]

The preliminary report was relatively modest in scope, since the commission's major recommendations would be presented in the final report the following April. The reaction was favorable, if somewhat subdued. Members of the National Advisory Mental Health Council were "generally satisfied," although they some expressed reservations. Jack R. Ewalt, who had directed the JCMIH between 1955 and 1961, was concerned that the PCMH had relied too much on public hearings for input. Such hearings, he noted, tended "to get people who have fish to peddle." Charles Kiesler, executive officer of the American Psychological Association, was critical of the dominance of consumer influence and would have preferred more "technical people" on the task panels. Bertram Brown, director of the NIMH, noted that the report was favorably received at his agency. He believed that the deinstitutionalization issue was well handled, the boundary issue less well. Brown was pleasantly surprised and pleased with the recommendations dealing with manpower training and research funding, although he thought that the latter did not go far enough. The sharpest criticisms came from E. Fuller Torrey, a psychiatrist who specialized in dealing with schizophrenia and mood disorder, which he believed to have a biological foundation. In a piece in *Psychology Today*, Torrey offered a harsh view of the preliminary report, which he regarded as "strictly Neolithic" because it transformed problems such as poverty and discrimination into mental health problems. The commission erred by largely neglecting the plight of people with severe mental disorders and supporting instead a national strategy for the prevention of mental illness and the promotion of mental health. "With everything except crabgrass defined as a mental-health problem, I, for one, certainly do not want anyone developing a 'national strategy.'" Bryant replied in an angry letter to the editor, but it was never published.[45]

Between October 1977 and January 1978 the commission held three two-day meetings during which it received and discussed the reports of the various task panels. The ensuing deliberations revealed that members were confronted with extraordinarily complex problems that grew out of both a global agenda that had no clear boundaries and the involvement of multiple interest groups with concerns that were not easily reconciled. It was quite feasible to consider the varied analyses and recommendations of a single panel. But it was questionable whether any group, professional or lay, could absorb the findings and recommendations of two dozen task panels and then develop a coherent final report. Further complicating the commission's deliberations was the fact that panels sometimes offered contradictory advice.

The October meeting was revealing. Six task panel coordinators provided interim reports dealing with community support systems, the family, public attitudes and media promotion of mental health, the CMHC program, legal and ethical issues, and manpower concerns. Their reports were complex and included numerous recommendations. The task panel on community support systems dealt with schools, religious organizations, the workplace, neighborhood organizations, and self-help and mutual aid groups. Its members were concerned with the ways in which such support groups could assist individuals with "normal wholistic [sic] personal development as well as coping with the stresses of mental illness," and how these groups could be linked with traditional mental health models. The panel on the family suggested that rather than treating individual pathology, the commission should focus on the reduction of societal pathology "by strengthening normal socializing agencies, with the family as the cornerstone of the system." The panel on the CMHC program was strongly supportive, but noted the absence of mechanisms to pick up patients discharged from state institutions, the fact that children and the elderly were underserved, and the failure of federal oversight. The group dealing with legal and ethical issues identified no fewer than nine problem areas, including a patient bill of rights, advocacy, financial assistance, confidentiality, the role of professionals, guardianship and custody, zoning, education, and mental health services to prisoners. The panel on manpower dealt with such issues as maldistribution, staffing, services to underserved groups, utilization of personnel, role blurring and role differentiation, and the federal role in manpower development.[46]

The December meeting was similar; six panels provided detailed summaries of their deliberations. The report of the Task Panel on Organization and Structure of Mental Health Services was in many respects typical. Its members attempted to develop a model that looked at the clustering of organizationally related structures in connection with three constituent groups: consumers, providers, and social institutions. In so doing they identified a series of theoretical categories.

> The categories "promotion" and "prevention" relate to a positive approach to mental health rather than the treatment of mental illness. "Identification" involves linking people who have problems but who do not necessarily need professional assistance into a natural environment. . . ."Intervention, Growth, Education, Restoration" lists a variety of growth services. "Crisis Stabilization" is self-explanatory, psychopathology and role performance used to be considered the major methods of treatment, but now we understand that psychopathology and social integration need to be looked at together. . . . "Collaboration/Coordination" and "Case Management" refer to the assistance consumers need now that emphasis has been moved from institutionalization to deinstitutionalization of mental patients.[47]

In the ensuing discussion Allen expressed concern. "How do you get from a theoretical place to what we have in reality?" She had doubts about the model's internal consistency as well as the absence of alternative models. In her eyes fragmentation was the major shortcoming of the mental health system. "It is impossible to negotiate the mental health system without four or five advocates, at least." Her pragmatic concerns stood in sharp contrast to the panel members' theoretical emphasis. The reports of the other task panels, which included planning, media promotion, legal and ethical issues, rural mental health, and prevention, posed similar kinds of problems because of their breadth. Albee's presentation on the important role of prevention, for example, drew support.[48] Cabranes, however, was less impressed. "How do you avoid the criticism," he asked, "that the expansive definition of mental health used by the Commission and the interest in prevention combine to make the Commission one that in effect would restructure society and speak not to physical but to social, political, and economic health?" Cabranes insisted that it was mandatory to develop a clear sense of what was meant by "prevention," the agencies involved, and the functional limits of the mental health system.[49]

The January meeting was even more frenetic. Over a two-day period the commission listened to briefings from twenty-two task and subtask panels, each providing multiple recommendations. The Task Panel on the Family, for example, reported that its objective was to examine the relationship of the family and the mental health of its members, and "to explore ways that public policies can enhance the ability of families to prevent emotional and mental disorders, to cope effectively with disorders when they occur, and in general to enable family members to live satisfying and socially useful lives." In addition, it wanted to develop programs that enhanced the ability "of neighborhoods, schools, communities, churches, places of recreation and of work, to nurture human potential, prevent stress, and manage resources well in time of crisis." Its ninety-three recommendations led the commissioners to suggest that they be translated into specific statutory and regulatory proposals. Nor was the presentation by the task panel on the family unique. Other panels—including those dealing with special populations, financing, research, personnel, deinstitutionalization, therapy and rehabilitation—made equally extensive and complex presentations.[50]

By early 1978 the task panels had completed their work. Their reports were lengthy and global in scope insofar as their analyses and recommendations were concerned: they filled 2,140 pages in three large volumes included as appendices to the commission's final report. The shortest was 10 pages; the longest 387 pages.[51] Indeed, their length, to say nothing about the number of individuals involved in their preparation, ensured diversity rather than unity. The constraints of time and the external obligations of the PCMH commissioners raised doubts about their ability to absorb the findings and recommendations of so many groups.

The task panel reports were heterogeneous in character. The first report, "The Nature and Scope of the Problems," stressed the need for data on prevalence and incidence (including data on such specific syndromes as schizophrenia and depression), location of patients, shifts in the locus of care, and occurrence of illness by life stages (childhood, adulthood, and old age). General health policy in the United States focused on chronic diseases with high mortality (cancer and heart disease). Often ignored were such mental disorders as depression, which had a high morbidity and a potential mortality by suicide. These disorders, like many nonpsychiatric chronic diseases, required comprehensive services that included crisis intervention for acute episodes and continuing care where appropriate. The report therefore emphasized the importance of epidemiological research as a basis for framing health and mental health policies.[52]

The report dealing with special populations, covering nearly 400 pages, was by far the longest and most exhaustive. It discussed women and Asian/Pacific, black, Hispanic, and Native Americans, as well as Americans of European ethnic origin and those with various kinds of handicaps. These groups were selected because they were both overrepresented in mental health statistics and were under- or inappropriately served. Its members were also de facto second-class citizens. The report also noted that most of those who provided services and conducted research did not share the "unique perspective, value systems and beliefs of the group being served." Research had also been hampered by the paucity of data that differentiated individuals by race, ethnicity, sex, and physically handicapped conditions. Subpanels dealing with each group issued their own reports, which tended to stress the presence of discriminatory barriers and the need for policies that took into account unique group characteristics. Four other task panels dealt with the elderly, migrant and seasonal farmworkers, Vietnam War veterans, and rural residents. By breaking down the population into such groups and emphasizing the role of discrimination, the need for social reforms, and the importance of positive mental health policies, the task panels implicitly lost sight of individuals with severe and persistent mental illnesses. Rather than constituting a single identifiable group, they were placed into groups whose distinguishing characteristics had little to do with specific diagnostic categories.[53]

The panel dealing with legal and ethical issues offered forty-two recommendations. Above all, its members insisted on building a strong patients' rights and consumer perspective into any changes in the service system. Its specific recommendations covered diverse subjects, including compensatory education for handicapped children, employment, housing, guardianship, confidentiality, right to treatment issues, experimentation, commitment, and mental health issues affecting individuals accused or convicted of crimes.[54]

Several reports were general and vague. The panel dealing with organization and structure, for example, urged the creation of active programs that promoted mental health, prevention, early identification, crisis stabilization, and the restoration or maintenance of mentally impaired persons at their maximum level of functioning. Similarly, the reports dealing with community support programs, access and barriers to care, and deinstitutionalization, rehabilitation and long-term care, were brief and superficial. Even the panel dealing with costs and financing—surely critical issues—conceded that the divergent views of members "limited the possibility that . . . [their] report would present agreements on the causes and cures for the problems of mental health financing." Hence it simply identified areas that required attention, and expressed the hope that the commission would recommend a national policy with regard to mental health services.[55]

The panel assessing CMHCs was strongly supportive and rejected criticisms that the centers had played a limited role in prevention, services to populations at special risk, and services to the previously institutionalized. Conceding the existence of serious problems, its members noted that relatively meager funding had produced important positive results. Unless the PCMH recommended a change in the distribution of funds, nothing the panel could recommend regarding CMHCs would make a difference.[56]

Other panels emphasized the important role of the states and expressed the hope that a partnership could be forged to overcome the mistrust and confusion that existed between various levels of government. Panels on prevention, research, personnel, alternative mental health services, family support services, media promotion of mental health, and learning failures all contributed to an agenda with no definite boundaries. Finally, three liaison panels reported on issues relating to mental retardation, alcohol-related problems, and use and misuse of psychoactive drugs.[57]

Having held public meetings and received the task panel reports, the commission in mid-February began its final task, the drafting of a final report that would be delivered to the president by April 1978. Although there had been long discussions dealing with numerous issues, there was as yet no consensus among members as to what should be included. The preliminary work had been done and a foundation laid, but the task of finding common ground and defining appropriate priorities and policies remained unfinished.

Chapter 4

From Advocacy to Legislation

With the task panels' reports in hand, the commission now faced the herculean task of absorbing their findings and recommendations and preparing a final report to submit to President Carter by April 1978. The writing of the report was complicated by the fact that most of the members did not share the same priorities. The issues were also challenging and difficult. The panel reports were sufficiently complex that the task of translating their recommendations into a coherent policy document was formidable. Moreover, the time to finish the final report was short.

The members of the PCMH rarely were in direct conflict and generally agreed on major issues. Nevertheless, each had his or her own agendas. Conlan, for example, insisted that unemployment was "the cause of many, many mental health problems." "I will not be trapped into easing off on this issue by an accusation that I am a do-gooder," he added. Willie, by contrast, felt that "prevention ought to be one of the major legs of our final report." Long agreed with Willie when she noted that "it is unconscionable to allow mental-emotional disability to develop when we know ways to prevent it." Nevertheless, she felt that the report had to address other issues, including the role of the federal government, the relationship between physical and mental health, and the financing of services. Beigel pointed to the vast changes that had occurred since 1961, but insisted that "a *system* of services has not kept pace," in part because of the policies and procedures of federal, state, and local governments. In offering its recommendations, he added, the commission "should avoid giving too much emphasis to a single area (e.g. children, prevention, financing, etc.)." Allen remained a spokesperson for persons with severe and persistent mental disorders. The condition of many of these persons "do not offer evidence of marked improvement," claims to the contrary notwithstanding. She rejected the community–institution dichotomy in which the former was allegedly superior to the latter, and expressed no interest in the broader agenda so attractive to many of her colleagues. "My efforts are directed toward the improvement of conditions for patients who reside both in inpatient, hospital-type facilities and 'in the community,' whether they receive services or non-services, either voluntary or involuntary." Her singular focus sometimes annoyed both her colleagues and the staff. She "had an image of herself as a powerless individual," Danaceau recalled. "But she probably had as much impact on the report as anyone. She was very informed and could make her point . . . even though she felt she did not have the power that professionals did. She was very effective in getting what she wanted considered and often adopted." Bryant also felt that Allen was "an extraordinarily bright person who could articulate what was wrong with the system." But she made things very difficult because she "could stop all action ."[1]

The February meeting of the commission was designed to begin the process of writing the final report. To facilitate that work, about thirty-five individuals had convened several weeks earlier for three days at the Wingspread Conference Center in Wisconsin to prepare a draft that dealt with the delivery of services. The participants included Joseph English (coordinator), members of the five core panels on service delivery, and liaison staff. The draft was intended to serve as the basis for discussion within the commission.[2]

At Wingspread the participants agreed on two broad themes: the necessity of fulfilling the federal commitment to community mental health services with full citizen participation; and the need for a new place and a new priority for the chronically disabled. The first required the development of a capacity to provide services and ensure adequate financing. Nor was a unitary system desirable; states and communities could develop quite different models. The second involved community living alternatives and employment issues, the future of the state hospital, a partnership between all levels of government rather than an adversarial relationship, and a way of financing care for the chronically disabled.[3]

The multiplicity of voices complicated the preparation of an acceptable final report. Each of the commissioners as well as the task panels had agendas that often differed even if they were not in direct opposition. In the early stages commissioners were provided with draft statements. Their comments on the initial drafts ranged so widely that Danaceau, whose journalism background gave him a unique vantage point, suggested to Bryant that all of them be deliberately incorporated into the document, which would then be "unbelievably long and confusing." When presented with this draft, the commissioners agreed that Bryant and his associates should assume responsibility for preparing a coherent report, which would then serve as the basis for discussions. At the February and March meetings Bryant proved adept in working out language acceptable to all the commissioners. The result was a unanimous report without minority dissents.[4]

The final report avoided the task panels' excessive details and innumerable recommendations. Although Bryant and his colleagues did not ignore the panels' work, they chose to present their case in a manner that would make it accessible to as wide an audience as possible. Despite the progress made during the previous twenty-five years, the report noted that many individuals "who should have benefitted from these changes still receive inadequate care," notably persons with chronic mental illnesses, children, adolescents and older Americans. Rural areas in particular lacked services.[5]

The plight of persons with chronic mental illnesses was illustrative. Most areas lacked a broad range of services that provided food, shelter, social supports, and psychiatric and general health care. Those with chronic mental illnesses, which included a large number of patients discharged from state mental hospitals, lived in poorly maintained facilities or in nursing homes ill equipped to meet their needs. Furthermore, those services that did exist all but ignored the differing cultural and linguistic traditions of minorities, including African Americans, Hispanics, Asian and Pacific Island Americans, Native Americans, and Alaskan Natives. The 5 million seasonal and migrant farmworkers, many of whom belonged to ethnic minorities, were almost entirely excluded from mental health care. Children and adolescents, as well as the 23 million Americans over the age of sixty-five, suffered from "neglect, indifference, and abuse" and lacked access to services. Moreover, perhaps 25 percent of the population suffered from mild to moderate emotional disorders, including depression and anxiety, to say nothing about the 40 million physically handicapped Americans. But mental health problems, the report continued,

> cannot be defined only in terms of disabling mental illnesses and identified psychiatric disorders. They must include the damage to mental health associated with unrelenting poverty and unemployment and the institutionalized discrimination that occurs on the basis of race, sex,

class, age, and mental or physical handicaps. They must also include
conditions that involve emotional and psychological distress which do
not fit convenient categories of classification or service.[6]

The report affirmed a commitment to the goal of making high-quality mental health care at reasonable cost available to all who needed it. Its attain-
ment was by no means unrealistic; the problem was the gap between "what we
know should be done and what we do." To narrow the gap, the commission
offered a series of recommendations that focused on eight areas it considered
of major importance.

First, it supported the strengthening of personal and community supports.
Such networks played an indispensable role by assisting individuals through
emotional crises, thus preventing more serious disability. Too often professionals and agencies were uncomfortable with these support systems. The nation
could ill afford to ignore such resources, and the report emphasized the need to
strengthen links between these supports and formal mental health services.[7]

Second, the United States was in need of a responsible mental health service system that provided the most appropriate care in the least restrictive
setting. What was required was a federal program designed to encourage the
creation of new community mental health services, particularly in areas where
none existed or in places where they were inadequate. Such services had to
involve ethnic and racial minorities in planning as well as providing culturally
relevant services staffed with bilingual and bicultural personnel. Nor could a
humane system of care exist until the needs of individuals with chronic mental
illnesses were addressed. It was imperative, therefore, that a "National Priority
to Meet the Needs of People with Chronic Mental Illness" be established. The
report urged DHEW to develop a national plan for phasing down and, where
appropriate, closing large mental hospitals and allocating more resources for
comprehensive and integrated systems care that included community-based
services and the remaining small state hospitals. In turn, states had to develop
linkages between their mental hospitals and communities and create a case
management system. "Performance contacts" would stipulate the "mutual expectations, responsibilities, and commitments" of states and the federal government. Finally, evaluative mechanisms would be created to ensure that services
were achieving their objectives.[8]

Third, there was a pressing need to reform both public and private arrangements for the financing of mental health services. Any future national health
insurance program and all existing private and public programs had to include

benefits for emergency, outpatient, and inpatient care. The report called for the abolition of discriminatory provisions in the Medicare program and strengthening of the Medicaid program. Equally important, private insurers had to provide outpatient mental health benefits and eliminate disparities that favored general health benefits over mental health benefits. Since persons with chronic mental illnesses required decent housing, adequate nutrition, and other supportive services, the commission maintained that any new system had to recognize the need for social welfare, as distinct from medical, expenditures.[9]

The fourth recommendation related to personnel. It called for a redirection of federal policy to encourage mental health specialists to work in underserved areas, to increase the number of minority personnel, and to ensure that the training and knowledge of such personnel were suitable for the needs of those they served. Commission members were particularly troubled by the lack of individuals trained specifically to work with children, adolescents, and the elderly. Implementing these and other goals required federal resources and moderate increases in funding levels for training and planning.[10]

The fifth recommendation dealt with legal and human rights. Given the social ferment of the 1960s and 1970s, this subject could hardly be avoided. The commission supported a series of actions: (1) the creation of an advocacy system to represent mentally disabled individuals; (2) the prohibition of discrimination; (3) a requirement that the states review their civil commitment and guardianship laws to ensure that they contained procedural protections; (4) affirmation of the rights to treatment in the least restrictive setting, rehabilitation, and protection from harm, as well as the right to refuse treatment with appropriate procedures under which this right could be qualified. Further, it asked that individuals caught up in the criminal justice system have access to relevant mental health services.[11]

The final recommendations dealt with research, prevention, and the improvement of public understanding. In regard to research and training, the commission supported increased funding, but in regard to the problems posed by stigmatization and discrimination, its members conceded that the commission did not know how to resolve them. Better data about how people actually viewed mental illnesses and emotional problems were needed, if only because older surveys were taken when most patients were confined in remote state hospitals rather than living in the community. It called upon the media to help eliminate stereotypes and present more accurate information to the public.[12]

In "A Strategy for Prevention," the commission noted that the history of public health during the past hundred years provided "ample evidence that

programs designed to prevent disease and disorder can be effective and eco-
nomical." Yet the mental health field had not taken advantage of available
knowledge. Prevention strategies required knowledge of the groups at risk as
well as the factors that contributed to risk. Only then was it possible to assess
whether or not the reduction of risk would lower the rate of emotional disorders or mental illnesses. Possible avenues of study were the reduction of the
stressful effects of life crisis experiences "such as unemployment, retirement,
bereavement, and marital disruption due to death or other circumstances." It
was equally important to understand the nature of social environments. The
first priority, however, was the mental health of children, and the report underscored the importance of appropriate prenatal and perinatal care, day care
programs, and foster care as ways of preventing mental disability in later life.
The commission also supported the creation of a Center for Prevention within
the NIMH, with primary prevention (the elimination of the causes of mental
disorder or disability) as its first priority.[13]

The final report also included more than one hundred other major recommendations that affected the relations among not only federal, state, and local
government but also public and private agencies and such federal programs
as Medicare and Medicaid. In many ways the heterogeneous character of the
commission's work was influenced by a political climate in which debates and
agendas were shaped by the demands of groups that defined themselves in
terms of class, gender, ethnicity, and race. By that time neither the state mental
hospital system nor individuals with serious and persistent mental disorders
were at the center of the policy debates; the number of competing voices and
advocates for other groups had increased exponentially. The PCMH, therefore,
had to take into account the claims of groups with far broader social and economic agendas that often had only tangential relationships to the needs of people with severe mental illnesses.[14]

The final report was neither a blueprint for legislative action nor the ex-
pression of a specific group. The diversity of its recommendations could not
easily be translated into legislation. At best, it was a document, as Steven S.
Sharfstein observed, that had the potential to create some sort of consensus that
would eventually result in legislation. Virtually every point of view and every
constituency was represented. In this sense it was as much a political document
as it was a policy proposal. The commission, deputy director Gary Tischler
recalled, "sought a political middle ground and its attempt was to honor the
various constituencies through recommendations that provided something for

everyone."[15] The inclusiveness of the report was thus a source of strength as well as a source of weakness.

In April 1978 the commission's final report was delivered to President Carter. At a press conference Carter spoke of his support for the commission's recommendations and his appreciation that the report had called for only modest increases in funding and had not recommended the initiation of new programs. "We will," he stated, "emphasize the prevention of mental illness, the care for those who chronically suffer from mental illness, the training of additional personnel who are qualified to treat those who suffer from this illness, the better distribution of their services around the country and to communities which are not presently served, and additional research with a minimum of expenditure of American finances how we can better deal with this severe problem that our nation still experiences."[16]

The hope of every modern presidential commission is to turn the public's attention to an important problem while providing new policy initiatives designed to mitigate the prevailing difficulties. Unlike the commissions that had dealt with urban violence, assassinations, and racial friction, however, the problems posed by mental illnesses and health appeared less immediate and hence less pressing. To be sure, those individuals with serious and persistent mental disorders faced extraordinarily difficult lives as the locus of care shifted from mental hospitals to the community. For most other groups, however, the issues that professionals subsumed under mental health did not have an especially high priority. Indeed, the poor and elderly rarely defined their needs in terms of mental health.

Even during its existence, the commission found it extraordinarily difficult to generate publicity that would focus public attention on the problem of mental health. From time to time the press covered some of its activities, but not in a systematic way.[17] Nor did the presence of Rosalynn Carter provide more than basic legitimacy. Admittedly, her activities in the mental health arena received substantial attention. Yet, as one observer noted, "almost all of the coverage . . . has focused on her personal charm and the fact that she is a 'working First Lady'"; substantive reporting was lacking, and what was reported was sometimes misleading.[18] Efforts to get the media to report on mental health problems also met with little success. When NBC was preparing a special three-hour television documentary on health care in America scheduled for showing on January 4, 1978, it included no mention of mental health. Contacted by the commission staff, Earl Ubell, producer and writer, explained that mental health was excluded because the subject was "so broad and complex." Bryant expressed his disappointment at the decision in a letter to the president of NBC News. Mental health, he observed, "is after all *a* major, if not the major, component of general health when viewed from the perspective of people needing care, people providing care and dollar spent for care."[19]

Unlike the publicity received by the reports of the Warren and Kerner commissions, the reception of the PCMH final report was relatively subdued. The *Washington Post,* which had covered the commission's activities, provided a summary (as did *Science News*), whereas the *Wall Street Journal* gave only six lines to the report. Among psychiatric periodicals *Hospital & Community Psychiatry* included a lengthy description. Here and there isolated articles were published. Frank Riessman, editor of *Social Policy,* for example, observed that presidential commissions become significant "only if they converge with other major forces in the society." Most of the commission's recommendations, he added, would probably fall by the wayside. The one exception was the members' emphasis on the important role that the proliferating self-help mutual aid networks could play. Self-help, he concluded, could involve the participation of the consumer in a "direct service producing capacity," thus bridging the gap between the promise and practice of mental health professional services. Alvin L. Schoor, a social worker teaching at the Catholic University of America, was extremely critical of the focus on professional issues and the lack of attention to other problems. "To account for epidemic emotional disorder," he insisted, "one must deal with concepts like poverty, unemployment, discrimination, and alienation." Although the commission acknowledged these problems, it did nothing with them.[20]

The APA's response was somewhat mixed. Jack Weinberg, its president, wrote to President Carter hailing the report "as an important step toward forging a national policy and commitment for adequate care and treatment of the mentally disabled." His diplomatic letter emphasized the high priority given to the chronically disabled, the need to strengthen research efforts, and the significance of creating new partnerships of the public and private sectors in providing treatment. Weinberg's failure to mention many of the other recommendations was equally notable. At its annual convention in May, the APA's Ad Hoc Committee on the PCMH, chaired by Robert Gibson, sponsored a special session that gave panel participants a chance to offer their own critiques.

The general consensus was that the report "could have been worse." Robert J. Campbell, chair of the Joint Commission on Government Relations, was critical of the use of the concept of mental health, if only because little of the human condition could be excluded, as well as the failure to differentiate services for mental illness from issues of health and happiness. Donald Langsley, who had served on the task panel dealing with personnel, was somewhat more sanguine. He believed that the report represented an effort to reverse the erosion of the research capacity in mental health and increase the supply of psychiatrists. Gibson was critical of the commission's failure to specify the resources required for mental health care. "Unless one dealt quite forthrightly with these concerns," he added, "the report might not really have a radical impact."[21]

That the report drew little attention did not mean that it would be ignored. Shortly after receiving the report, President Carter directed DHEW secretary Califano to draft a law that would implement its recommendations. Califano in turn created an internal task force to identify and analyze the implications of the report and to propose legislation. On the advice of his staff, he directed that the proposed legislation concentrate on revising the CMHC Act and categorical mental health services. His staff believed that if the draft law attempted to address the comprehensive needs of persons with severe mental illnesses, Congress would be unlikely to act.[22]

By this time it was clear that the decentralized and uncoordinated mental health system was not providing integrated and comprehensive services to persons with severe and persistent mental illnesses, who were those with the greatest needs. Hence there was increasing interest in a systems approach that would forge links between the mental health system, on the one hand, and other health and human services, on the other. The presumption was that people with severe and persistent mental disorders required a range of life and social supports. The best-known effort to design an integrated program occurred at the University of Wisconsin in Madison. In the late 1960s Leonard Stein, Mary Ann Test, and others began to develop an integrated community mental health care program designed to assist patients to leave the hospital and live in the community. Out of this emerged the Training in Living project. Patients in the experimental program were taught coping skills and provided with housing, jobs, and social support services. Provision was made for ongoing monitoring, including crisis intervention, and—where possible—family members were involved in the program. The model that evolved over time deemphasized traditional office psychiatry and the use of professional facilities. Its central concern was with the provision of care to patients in the community and at their place of residence.[23] In 1977 the NIMH undertook a related effort when it launched its Community Support Program (CSP).[24]

In this context the DHEW task force on implementing the PCMH report began composing its recommendations, which took nearly eight months to complete. Its assignment was complicated by the absence of any clear programmatic consensus both without and within the government, to say nothing of leadership turnover in key positions. Gerald L. Klerman, a well-known psychiatrist, had only recently been appointed as the new administrator of the DHEW's Alcohol, Drug Abuse, and Mental Health Administration (AD-AMHA). Moreover, at the NIMH Herbert Pardes had just replaced Bertram Brown. Klerman, who headed the DHEW task force, had the unenviable task of developing implementation proposals and then guiding them through the various bureaucratic levels, beginning with the NIMH and ADAMHA. Beyond them, assistant secretaries for health, legislation, management and budget, planning and evaluation were involved, to say nothing of consultation with the Social Security Administration as well as a number of outside groups. Before being completed, the legislative draft went through six major revisions. Disagreements and differences were omnipresent, but the process was largely dominated by DHEW staff.[25]

The DHEW task force prepared a draft of a community mental health systems act as the means of implementing the letter and spirit of the PCMH's recommendations. The draft offered a detailed blueprint for legislative action. But its very inclusiveness—born out of a desire to please the different constituencies—resulted in a document that lacked cohesion and did not offer any clear vision to guide future policy. It called for a state–federal partnership that would improve state planning and management of mental health services. Such a partnership would facilitate the development of community services for unserved, underserved, and inappropriately served populations, including children and youth, the aged, persons with chronic mental disorders, racial and ethnic minorities, poor persons, and persons in rural areas. CMHCs would continue to receive federal funding. Institutionalization would be minimized and steps taken to ensure that those suffering from mental disorders or disability received care in the least restrictive setting possible. General health and mental health services would be integrated, and states encouraged to develop prevention programs. There would be incentives to increase the supply of professional personnel in unserved and underserved areas. Finally, the draft provided support for demonstration and pilot projects as well as evaluation and monitoring.[26]

In its report, the PCMH had supported the establishment of a national priority to meet the needs of those with chronic illnesses, and had called upon DHEW to develop a national plan. The DHEW task force, in turn, indicated that such a plan should be included in a report to the Congress. This recommendation was modified by department officials, who proposed instead that the secretary of DHEW appoint a task force to develop a "National Plan for the Chronically Mentally Ill." Other agencies (Departments of Labor, Housing and Urban Development, and Agriculture) would be represented in the formulation of such a plan, which would be completed within eighteen months.[27]

Even before completing its work, the DHEW group was sharply criticized. Robert Gibson emphasized several shortcomings. He pointed to the failure to address the substandard staff and environment in public mental hospitals, the lopsided nature of the patient rights section, the disregard of the need to ensure that funding followed patients from institutional to community settings, and the relative neglect of persons with chronic illness. Other groups, including state mental health program directors who were opposed to performance contracts and representatives of CMHCs fearful of a decline in funding, expressed reservations as well.[28]

In March 1979 a draft was sent to the White House and the Office of Management and Budget (a reflection of Carter's attempt to impose zero-based budgeting in the federal government). Because of his close relationship with Rosalynn Carter, Bryant was asked to review the draft legislation. He found the draft

> not exciting, it does not represent the bold new thrust in mental health that many hoped would come with the Carter Commission. Rather it is a sort of "fix-things-up" bill. (It does seek to "fix" a number of things that need repair!) I think the bill can be made far more exciting and attractive.
>
> The major mental health-related problem at the present, so far as public program and dollars are concerned, is the care of the chronically mentally ill—the "deinstitutionalized" population. The federal government's role in caring for this population is unclear. The bill offers the chance to clarify that role and to forge the necessary new partnerships with the states to implement a new national effort in this regard. That opportunity should not be missed.

Bryant's comments did not necessarily reflect a change of heart. Rather they suggested that once freed from the burden of running the PCMH and the need to satisfy multiple points of view and constituencies, he was able to focus on the core problem that had been subsumed by the commission's seemingly boundless agenda. The bill was returned to the DHEW task force, which sent a revised and acceptable version to the White House in April 1979.[29]

Following in the footsteps of John F. Kennedy, President Carter sent a message to Congress the following month accompanied by a draft of a "mental health systems" act. The very title of the legislation represented a subtle change; the original recommendation of the DHEW task force had employed "community" in its title. At the very outset Carter emphasized the creation of a new federal–state partnership that would ensure that "the chronically mentally ill no longer face the cruel alternative of institutionalization or inadequate care in the community." Summarizing the findings of his commission, he expressed the belief that the new legislation would encourage "the development of a comprehensive, integrated system of care designed to best serve the needs of the chronically mentally ill adults and children." The act's flexibility would also enable communities to provide services to a variety of underserved populations, including the elderly, racial and ethnic minorities, the poor, and rural residents.[30]

The draft act had six titles. Title I was directed toward the improvement of mental health services for adults and children with chronic mental illnesses, and promised federal funding to develop community-based systems. Title II and III offered grants to programs dealing with the prevention of mental illnesses and the improvement of state mental health systems. Title IV, the longest, offered grant funding to develop services for the underserved (particularly in areas lacking a CMHC), to integrate general health and mental health care, and to provide continuing support for CMHCs. Title V dealt with demonstration grants for states to develop pilot programs to administer federal grants. Title VI had two main parts. The first required states to develop a mental health plan that would identify needs and services and address the need to protect the rights of the mentally ill and handicapped. The second required mental health professionals receiving federal funding for a clinical traineeship to serve in an underserved area.[31]

The introduction of a draft law was only a beginning; passage of the final bill took nearly a year and a half. Congressional inaction was by no means the result of disinterest or preoccupation with other issues. Rather, there was no consensus on mental health policy. Deinstitutionalization—whatever its meaning—was coming under widespread criticism. The decision by the *Milbank Memorial Fund Quarterly* to devote an entire issue to the subject was indicative of the policy void. Deinstitutionalization, concluded one of the contributors to this issue, failed

> to provide even minimally adequate aftercare and community support services anywhere in the nation. Instead, the rhetoric of deinstitutionalization seems to mask a brutal political and economic reality—the general abandonment of mentally disabled people who have been further debilitated, mentally and physically, by institutionalization. Evidence indicates that the new policy has brought with it a new set of mental health problems, including massive numbers of people needing rehospitalization; gross inadequacies in community resources for aftercare and rehabilitation; large-scale scandal, exploitation, and abuse in the new industry of operating community facilities; increased drug and alcohol dependency among released patients; and an apparent social and psychological decay among patients released into nursing homes, adult homes, or welfare hotels.[32]

By this time a number of interest groups had formed, each with a different agenda. The concerns of CMHCs, for example, differed from those of state officials. The original legislation creating such centers bypassed state governments; the result was continuing friction between the federal government and CMHCs on the one hand and state mental health authorities on the other. It had become equally clear that CMHCs had contributed little to a reduced resident rate in state hospitals, and that many deinstitutionalized individuals faced major problems in the community. The very role of CMHCs in the mental health system remained an open question.[33] Moreover, the proliferation of the mental health professions had created other constituencies having either a tangential or no relationship to persons with serious and persistent mental illnesses. To forge a consensus that would result in new legislation would not be easy.

The daunting task of building a broad-based coalition did not in any way inhibit Rosalynn Carter. She saw the completion of the work of the PCMH as merely a beginning, and consequently continued her advocacy work. Two months before her husband's message and submission of a draft law to the Congress, she began a campaign designed to spur congressional action. On February 7, 1979, she appeared before Senator Edward M. Kennedy's Subcommittee on Health and Scientific Research. Her presence was unusual. The last First Lady to testify before Congress had been Eleanor Roosevelt, who had appeared on behalf of the poor, homeless, and underserved in 1942, and as a private citizen in 1955 and 1962. When Rosalynn Carter appeared before the subcommittee, it was clear that her involvement with the PCMH had altered her perspective. Conceding that CMHCs had made "enormous contributions," she nevertheless acknowledged that they had not met the needs of special populations. Like Bryant, she emphasized that the problems of persons with chronic disorders "dramatically point up critical weaknesses in our present system of care—the lack of adequate planning, poor coordination between federal, state and local programs, blurred lines of responsibility and accountability, treatment programs dictated by reimbursement mechanisms rather than patient needs." To be sure, she accepted many of the other recommendations presented in the PCMH's final report. Nevertheless, her focus on persons with chronic mental illnesses was suggestive of the changes in her views since her first involvement in mental health in Georgia.[34]

Her testimony struck a sympathetic chord with the members of the subcommittee, both Democrat and Republican. Indeed, Edward Kennedy noted that for many persons with mental illnesses "the system of mental health care remains a national disgrace," and he looked forward to working with the administration in an effort to improve conditions.[35] In a subsequent contribution to the *Milbank Memorial Fund Quarterly,* however, he criticized the DHEW draft legislation. The original CMHC Act of 1963, he claimed, was premised on creating "an integrated system of services utilizing federal, state, public, and private resources." That vision, however, had proved "elusive." Although Kennedy's description of the 1963 legislation was in error, his claim that there were two independent and uncoordinated service systems (CMHCs and state mental hospitals) was accurate. The PCMH's report, he conceded, was "thorough and incisive," but the "modest" legislative proposal that followed did not go far enough in dealing with the basic problem; it merely begged the question of expanding services and focused instead on better management of existing meager resources. The overriding need was "for strong, federally financed support for programs in housing, income maintenance, and other rehabilitation services," which in turn required changes in Titles XVIII, XIX, and XX of the Social Security Act.[36] Yet the DHEW draft all but ignored the critical role of these titles in any revamped system.

In late May 1979 the draft bill submitted by DHEW to President Carter was introduced in the Senate (S1177) and the House of Representatives (HR4156). That the concept of mental health had the ability to attract a variety of constituencies was evident in the deliberations of the House, where a second piece of legislation (HR3986) was introduced amending the CMHC Act to provide further research and services to victims of rape. In May and June both Senate and House subcommittees held public hearings on the president's draft legislation, and the latter also included in its deliberations the bill dealing with rape.

The political context at that time was anything but ideal. Kennedy, who chaired the subcommittee responsible for mental health legislation, had become alienated from the Carter administration, which he believed was abandoning his party's liberal foundations. As Carter's popularity in the polls dipped, Kennedy began to prepare to challenge the president in the forthcoming primaries. The relationship between both men became increasingly tense. The firing of DHEW secretary Califano in July 1979 exacerbated the situation, if only because of Kennedy's belief that Carter was seeking a scapegoat for his own shortcomings.[37]

Only two months earlier, Kennedy's subcommittee had held two hearings. Califano was the first witness, and he agreed that there was a pressing need to coordinate Titles XVIII, XIX, and XX. He also expressed implicit criticism of CMHCs because of the absence of linkages to deal with individuals discharged from mental hospitals. Although his testimony met with general accolades, Kennedy suggested that the laudable goals of the draft law were not matched by sufficient resources. Other committee members also expressed reservations. Senator Richard S. Schweiker feared that targeting services to specific groups might undermine the goal of comprehensive services accessible to all. Senator Jacob K. Javits believed that the draft bill failed to adequately take into account the plight of discharged patients with chronic mental illnesses. "Not only are these people not receiving needed mental health services," he observed, "but their most basic living needs are not being addressed."[38]

The testimony of those who followed Califano was hardly friendly. Although there was general agreement on the need for creative mental health legislation, the Senate hearings demonstrated that strong and determined opposition to the draft legislation might very well result in its defeat. Supporters of CMHCs were disturbed by the absence of a firm commitment to the program. Others believed that the draft did not address the problem of creating a coherent working relationship among the three levels of government. Some argued that states—which supplied more mental health dollars than the federal government—did not have an adequate voice in determining how federal dollars were spent. Civil rights advocates were disturbed by the absence of a patients' bill of rights. And many decried the bill's failure to address the needs of racial and ethnic minorities.[39]

The absence of a consensus on the shape of mental health policy was evident throughout the hearings. Hilda Robbins, national president of the Mental
Health Association, expressed surprise and puzzlement about Califano's comments about CMHCs and discharged patients. She conceded that centers bore
some responsibility, but insisted that they represented an "infinitely better"
system than the old state hospital approach. John Wolfe, executive director
of the National Council of Community Mental Health Centers, regarded the
draft as an effort to shift total responsibility from the federal government to the
states. Admitting that centers did not always provide services to minorities,
the elderly, and deinstitutionalized patients, he pointed to the lack of resources and "turf fights" between a variety of agencies and professions. Robert E.
McGarrah from the American Federation of State, County, and Municipal Employees (AFSCME), argued that deinstitutionalization had very adverse effects
on mental hospital personnel, and pointed out that DHEW had failed to address retraining and job placement despite federal legislation mandating such
action. CMHCs, he added, should be required to follow discharged patients and
ensure that they receive care and support services. Paul R. Friedman, director of the Mental Health Law Project, emphasized the conflict between states,
which had responsibility to deliver services, and advocates seeking to protect
patients. Eight other witnesses testified on behalf of such underserved populations that included African Americans, Hispanics, Pacific Asians, women, and
victims of rape.[40]

A number of professional organizations sent representatives or submitted
position papers. The National Association of State Mental Health Program Directors, an organization long at odds with the federal government since the passage of the CMHC Act of 1963, did not believe that the legislation adequately
addressed the critical issues of coordination and integration, and argued that
it perpetuated two distinct systems, CMHCs and state mental hospitals. The
organization was particularly critical of the emphasis on state demonstration
projects. Careful analysis, it added in blunt terms, "will show that the capacity
of state government to manage a mental health system is *not open to debate.*"
Gary Vandenbos, representing the American Psychological Association and
the Association for the Advancement of Psychology, argued that there was a
need for a stronger emphasis on prevention, criticized the recommendation
that more primary care providers be trained in mental health, and pointed to
the critical need for more fully trained mental health practitioners. Lee Macht,
the spokesperson of the APA, supported "the concept and framework" of the
bill, but was critical of many of its provisions. The bill "did not adequately

emphasize the need for community support systems for the longterm patient in the Community." Its funding levels were inadequate; it failed to incorporate changes in Medicaid, Medicare, SSDI, and housing supports; and it did little to further the integration of mental health services into general hospitals. Several organizations, including the American Hospital Association, the American Nurses' Association, the American Occupational Therapy Association, stressed problems unique to their membership.[41]

The hearings before the House subcommittee were even more divided and contentious than their Senate counterpart. During Califano's testimony, Tim Lee Carter, a Kentucky representative and physician, suggested that the bill lacked oversight mechanisms. Two other subcommittee members questioned funding levels. Representative William E. Dannemeyer wanted to know where the additional $50 million would come from, and implied that Califano did not believe there was a limit on the level of taxation. Representative Phil Gramm of Texas was critical of federal spending and maintained that the health arena could benefit from greater competition.[42]

Some of the same individuals and organizational representatives appearing before the Senate subcommittee were present at the House hearings as well. Advocates of minorities and underserved populations repeated their testimony. Mildred Mitchell-Bateman, who had been a PCMH commissioner, reiterated the theme that children and preventive interventions deserved higher priorities. Others insisted that the legislation was deficient because it did not address the need for adequate resources. Conflict between representatives of CMHCs and state mental health authorities also persisted. John Ambrose, president of the National Council of Community Mental Health Centers, declared that provisions of the draft legislation "do not amount to a mid-course correction but establish a fragmented system and weaken the existing system of mental health care in this country." Youlon D. Savage from the National Association of Social Workers declared that the most pressing need was not to create more "specialty programs," but rather to increase the number of CMHCs. Anthony Carnevale of AFSCME pointed to the ineffectiveness of deinstitutionalization as a policy. Nor, he testified, was the draft legislation impressive; it did not provide adequate funding, and it gave resources to CMHCs that did not treat individuals with chronic mental disorders. He also repeated the charge that DHEW failed to meet statutory obligations to provide protection for mental hospital employees adversely affected by deinstitutionalization. Representing the National Association of State Mental Health Program Directors, George A. Zitnay was supportive of the PCMH's recommendations, but lambasted the draft bill. "In the

torturous course of developing Federal legislation through Federal Agencies,"
he declared, "much of the President's Commission's intentions suffered from a
metamorphosis that made the final product a fragmented, uncoordinated non-
system of projects, impossible for the State mental health agencies to support."
The House subcommittee hearing was made even more complex by the simultaneous presence of the draft bill dealing with victims of rape.[43]

More than two years had passed since the Carter administration had created the
PCMH. In spite of the commission's report, the general consensus on the need
for change, and the continued involvement of Rosalynn Carter and the DHEW
bureaucracy, the prospects for the passage of the mental health systems act appeared dim. The testimony before both subcommittees had revealed significant
policy differences between constituent groups that were not easily reconciled.
The firing of Califano only a month after the Senate and House subcommittee
hearings as well as other changes among agency staff made the prospects of
passage even more problematic. The appointment of Patricia Roberts Harris
as DHEW secretary introduced a measure of stability, if only by reducing the
tension that had prevailed between the White House and Califano. Under her
administration a team was formed to begin work on developing a modified
legislative draft that took into account the disparate concerns of the numerous
interest groups. The hope, according to Sharfstein, was to build "a coalition of
mental health interests strong and durable enough to get the legislation through
the rigors of subcommittee review and revision."[44]

Initially the Senate subcommittee staff began to rewrite the legislation without consulting any of the interested parties. The completion of an initial draft
in October 1979 was met with angry opposition from all constituent groups,
who threatened to oppose the rewrite. An agreement to consult widely averted
a crisis. The legislation went through seven rewrites before the full Committee
on Labor and Human Resources reported the bill out the following spring. Each
draft, according to Sharfstein, "represented an increasingly broader statement
of agreement if not actual consensus among the groups and the administration
. . . [and] created an increasingly cohesive coalition" that played an important
role in the eventual passage of the legislation.[45]

The bill that emerged in the Senate was quite different than the original
DHEW draft. It included a commitment to the continuation and expansion of
CMHCs, although it permitted other local and state agencies to apply for funds

to provide mental health services to a variety of groups. But it also created an extraordinarily complex process of combined local, state, and federal planning and management. It incorporated as well a patients' bill of rights and advocacy program, stronger employee protection overseen by the Department of Labor, greater attention to individuals with chronic mental illnesses, more services for rape victims, and the creation of an associate director for minority concerns and the establishment of an administrative unit "for the prevention of mental illness and the promotion of mental health," both within the NIMH. The new draft, the committee maintained, provided "clearer and better lines of responsibility for providing mental health services at all levels of government" as well as developing "a closer partnership between the Federal and State governments and a better working relationship between Federal, State, and local government and community groups." It also offered additional resources to care for the deinstitutionalized patient. In sum, the Senate bill promised a sharp expansion in services and resources.[46]

In the House subcommittee a somewhat different situation prevailed. The members of that committee, more so than their Senate counterparts, were directly involved in the legislative process. Henry A. Waxman, a liberal Democrat from California, wanted to ensure that underserved populations had access to CMHCs, whereas Tim Lee Carter, the ranking Republican from Kentucky, was committed to a more comprehensive approach and feared further fragmentation. A number of members in both the subcommittee and the full committee, moreover, were unhappy with the entire bill. During the June hearings members had been impressed by the claim that CMHCs were not meeting the needs of individuals with chronic mental illnesses. Consequently, the subcommittee decided to hold two additional hearings, the first dealing with the care of patients with chronic mental illnesses and the second with CMHCs.[47]

In October 1979 the subcommittee held a hearing to examine community supports for persons with chronic disorders. Some individuals offered testimony that focused on successful community programs such as Fountain House in New York City. But others, including John A. Talbott, Ann Klein (commissioner, New Jersey Department of Human Services), and Martha Hodge (coordinator of Georgia's community support projects), expressed considerable misgivings about the current state of affairs. Talbott pointed out that rates of institutionalization had not changed since 1950. The difference was that the percentage of individuals in nursing homes had tripled. What had taken place was transinstitutionalization rather than deinstitutionalization. "We need," he added,

a resolution of the fragmentation between Federal, State, and local governments; an end to the fragmentation between governmental agencies
at all levels . . . which all have different regulations and different eligibility; full civil rights in housing and education and vocational areas,
and full access to quality medical and psychiatric care; and an orienta-
tion toward care, not cure, toward maintenance in the community, and
toward asylum for some residual population.[48]

Klein was critical of the administration's draft bill because it failed to address the problems faced by individuals with chronic mental disorders. If their
needs were not met in the community, she observed, "we will[,] once again,
be taking care of them in some sort of institutional setting, and these settings,
if they are to be decent, are going to be very, very expensive, and if they are
not very, very expensive, they are going to be, again, a blot against the State's
record." Hodge had major reservations about CMHCs. Their staffs preferred individual psychotherapy and were not trained to deal with highly disabled persons. States had very little authority over CMHCs, which lacked connections
with public mental hospitals. The mission of CMHCs, moreover, had become
unfocused and "grandiose"; they were expected to do more and more with
less and less.[49] At a second hearing several months later, Sharfstein, director of
NIMH's Division of Mental Health Service Programs, provided both a description and an analysis of the CMHC program.[50]

In early May of 1980 the House subcommittee sent its own draft to the
Committee on Interstate and Foreign Commerce. The draft was more modest
in scope than its Senate counterpart, although it was by no means a rejection
of the administration bill. Nevertheless, there was more opposition in the full
committee. Six out of the forty-two members filed a dissenting report. They
conceded that the results of the creation of CMHCs "ranged from satisfactory
to spectacular." Had the program stopped there, "it would have been one of
the more inspired efforts in federal legislation." The new legislation would
substantially increase costs. The greatest need, they insisted, was to balance
the budget. Moreover, the new legislation did not resolve the problem of fragmentation. Finally, the bill would start the government upon an entirely new
project designed to prevent mental illness, a move that was "frightening from
both a philosophical and a fiscal point of view."[51]

On July 24 the Senate began debate on the legislation. A coalition of mental
health advocacy groups had succeeded in their efforts to persuade the Committee of Labor and Human Resources to include a patients' bill of rights. The APA,

which was sometimes at odds with legal advocates preoccupied with patient rights, was opposed to many of its provisions, which it felt would compromise quality medical and psychiatric care. When the bill reached the floor of the House, opposition to this provision emerged. Senator Robert Morgan of North Carolina introduced a substitute amendment that "it was the sense of Congress" that each state should review and revise its laws to ensure that patients received the protection and services that they required. The rights of patients, in other words, would be determined by states rather than by the federal government. Despite opposition from some legal scholars and mental health advocacy groups, Kennedy was forced to yield because of a threatened filibuster. The amended bill then passed by an overwhelming vote.[52]

A month later the House took up the version of the bill reported by its Committee on Interstate and Foreign Commerce. This legislation lacked a patients' bill of rights. After a debate and the adoption of some relatively minor amendments, the bill was adopted by a vote of 277 to 15 (with 140 members not voting) on August 22.[53]

The stage was now set for the Senate and House to reconcile the differences in their respective bills. At a three-hour session in Senator Kennedy's office in September, members from both branches of Congress managed to resolve two major differences.[54] The first concerned the absence of regulations dealing with the protection of hospital employees who were in danger of losing their jobs when hospitals were closed. Because AFSCME had earlier threatened to oppose the legislation, the Senate bill acceded to its demands and assigned responsibility for promulgating protective regulations to the Department of Labor. Grants for services to individuals with chronic disorders could be used for job placement and retraining for employees of inpatient facilities. Waxman, chair of the House subcommittee, was opposed to this provision. A compromise version required the secretary of health and human services (DHSS) to issue regulations describing the arrangements each state mental health authority must have in effect to protect adversely affected employees. The secretary of labor had to concur with these regulations. Failure by state authorities to comply could result in financial penalties.[55]

The second major point of dispute revolved around the patients' bill of rights. The Senate bill included a "sense of Congress" provision that each state was required to have a system to protect the rights of individuals with mental illnesses; those that chose not to adopt such protections would be ineligible to receive funds for community mental health services. The House draft, however, had not included such a provision. In the end the Senate version was accepted

by members of both branches, but only after the deletion of the section providing for penalties for states that had no protective legislation. In general, the conference committee, with some exceptions, reported out a bill on September 22
that was closer to the more expansive Senate version. Within days both chambers had accepted the conference report and approved the legislation, which
was signed into law on October 7 at a ceremony at a northern Virginia CMHC.
Senator Kennedy, who was present at the signing, remarked that the bill was a
"living monument" to Rosalynn Carter's "commitment and to her concern."[56]

Enacted two and a half years after the creation of the PCMH, the Mental Health
Systems Act was an extraordinarily complex and contradictory piece of legislation. Its passage had involved a number of interest groups that were sometimes at odds and often had divergent goals. Supporters of CMHCs were determined to protect their own interests. State mental health officials, a group
that had responsibility for overseeing the welfare of persons with severe and
persistent mental illnesses both within and without institutions, were seeking
to regain some of the authority they had lost since the passage of the act of
1963. Advocates for ethnic and racial minorities, children, the elderly, victims
of rape, and other underserved groups wanted to ensure their Constituents'
access to services. Various professional groups and hospital employees each
had their own agenda. In addition, the act was passed at a time when infla-
tion and rising health care costs had created a climate that made it difficult to
introduce new initiatives that involved large expenditures. Under these circumstances it was hardly surprising that the legislation that finally emerged
lacked a central focus.

The provisions of the Mental Health Systems Act reflected the ambiguities
and contradictions that had been characteristic of mental health policy during
the preceding two decades. The act pointed to the achievements since 1963 in
making community mental health facilities available. But it also noted the failure to provide services to a variety of groups and the absence of a coordinated
system. The intent of the legislation was to create new opportunities and initiatives. The federal government would continue to play a leading role by using
grant funding as a catalyst for change while simultaneously creating a new relationship with states designed to overcome the prevailing policy fragmentation.
The act reaffirmed the priority for community mental health services, particularly for underserved groups such as individuals with chronic mental illnesses,
children and youth, the elderly, ethnic and racial minorities, women, the poor,

and rural residents. It emphasized planning and accountability and mandated "performance contracts" as a condition for federal funding, the creation of new intergovernmental relationships, and closer links between the mental health and the general health care systems.[57]

The legislation provided grants for a variety of purposes: to CMHCs that had not received federal funding; to state mental health authorities, CMHCs, or other entities providing services to persons with chronic mental illnesses, severely disturbed children and adolescents, elderly persons, and other priority populations; to health care centers to provide mental health services; to training and retraining programs for displaced employees; to programs for the prevention of mental illness and promotion of mental health; and to state mental health authorities to plan and develop mental health services programs and coordinate them with other federal programs providing services to persons with mental illnesses (for example, the various titles of the Social Security Act as well as legislation dealing with other disabled groups). Some of its provisions were designed to restore the balance that the original CMHC Act of 1963 lacked. The states' mental health authorities were given more power to review applications for community services. The NIMH was required to create a mental health prevention unit. Funds were dispensed through "performance contracts" in order to ensure accountability. The law included a relatively weak provision dealing with a patients' bill of rights and advocacy programs, as well as titles dealing with rape prevention and the control and protection of employees adversely affected by the introduction of new policies.[58]

In many ways the Mental Health Systems Act mirrored the contradictions and inconsistencies of the nation's mental health system. It recognized that the traditional policy of hospitalizing persons with chronic mental illnesses in long-stay and remote institutions was no longer acceptable, and that care and treatment in a community setting was the preferred policy. The latter required not only psychiatric services but a variety of social support services for a population whose illness also created dependency. While assigning the highest priority to individuals with chronic mental illnesses, the legislation also recognized the claims of various other groups whose needs were quite different, including children and adolescents, the elderly, rural residents, and victims of rape. The absence of new resources and vague generalizations about the kinds of services required, however, raised doubts about the legislation's effectiveness.

Since the legislation mirrored the demands of multiple interest groups, it is not surprising that it offered prescriptions for action that reflected quite different concerns. As Sharfstein noted, in order to make it through the congressional gauntlet, the legislation "had to give a little something to everyone and as a result became unusually complex." Older CMHCs were criticized because they had not responded to the needs of vulnerable populations, yet the act authorized funding for areas that had not received grants. Although the legislation anticipated the creation of an integrated effort at the local level, it created ten new categorical programs, each with its own constituency.[59]

Some of the legislation's provisions reflected ideology rather than empirical data, notably the provisions dealing with the prevention of mental illnesses and the promotion of mental health. Their popularity reflected in part a faith in human agency, that disease was not inevitable and could be avoided by conscious and purposive actions. In fact, the prevention of mental illnesses and promotion of mental health were little more than attractive slogans. Given that neither the etiology nor the pathology of mental illnesses was understood, how could strategies be developed that would prevent such disorders and promote health? The absence of any data demonstrating the effectiveness of preventive and promotion strategies did not, however, act as a deterrent.

Even more important, how could individuals with serious mental illnesses in the community negotiate with programs administered by independent agencies? To be sure, the act implicitly recognized the critical role of federal entitlement programs. Yet it made no systematic provisions to ensure that individual needs would be addressed by the agencies administering these programs, each of which had different missions and concerns. Despite paying homage to the need to integrate services and to strengthen the regulatory role of state mental health authorities, the act did little to overcome the fragmentation characteristic of the mental health field.

The Mental Health Systems Act had hardly become law when its provisions were rendered moot. The inauguration of Ronald Reagan in January 1981 led to an immediate reversal of policy. Preoccupied with reducing both taxes and federal expenditures and creating a "new federalism," the new administration called for a 25 percent cut in federal funding. More important, it proposed the elimination of federal mental health programs and the substitution in its place of a single block grant to the states that would carry few restrictions and would include no policy guidelines. Reagan's original proposal would have left a variety of services—psychiatric and medical—to compete with each other for state allocations. Waxman, however, emerged as the staunchest defender of health programs and prevented such a consolidation. Nevertheless, in the summer of 1981 the Omnibus Budget Reconciliation Act was signed into law. This legislation effectively ended the federal CMHC program. Under the act's provisions, the federal government provided a block grant to states for mental health services and substance abuse, although at levels of about 75 to 80 percent of what they would have received under the Mental Health Systems Act. The states had considerable leeway in expending their allocations, which meant that they would be faced with pressures to distribute funds to many different groups. With a few exceptions—notably the patients' bill of rights—the Mental Health Systems and CMHC acts were repealed, thus seemingly diminishing the direct role of the federal government in mental health. Although state mental health authorities gained somewhat more power, the issue of fragmentation remained as pressing as ever, if only because there was no effort to integrate federal entitlement with state mental health programs.[60] The transfer and decentralization of authority merely exacerbated the existing tensions, as federal support was reduced at precisely the same time that the states were faced with a variety of social and economic problems that increased their fiscal burdens.

By 1981 it had become clear that the effort to create a more coherent and integrated mental health system for persons with serious and persistent mental illnesses had fallen short of its goals. The PCMH might have laid out a blueprint for the future, but the very composition of its membership led to deliberations that focused on the needs of multiple interest groups. In the judgment of David Mechanic, coordinator of the Task Panel on the Nature and Scope of the Problems, the PCMH "functioned in an atmosphere of much greater fiscal constraints and with many more well-developed constituencies anxious to protect their interests." As a result the report was overly general, provided no clear direction among competing constituencies, and failed to face "the tough question of financial priorities." Aware of the difficulty of balancing competing interests, he would have preferred focusing directly on the needs of the most severely mentally ill. "While these received much attention, other vague concepts such as prevention received equal play. In endorsing everything, the report offered no clear course of action."[61]

In the short run the PCMH appeared to have relatively little influence on the evolution of mental health policy. Yet serendipity is often an unrecognized force in human affairs. This is particularly true of the section in the final report calling for the establishment of a national priority and a national plan to meet the needs of individuals with chronic mental illnesses. As a result of this recommendation, the DHEW task force charged with drafting a law proposed that the secretary of the agency appoint a group to develop a "National Plan for the Chronically Mentally Ill." While the legislation was working its way through Congress, Patricia Harris appointed an internal group in August 1979 to prepare such a plan.

Completed in December 1980, the plan began with the assumption that individuals with severe and disabling mental illnesses could "live in their home communities even during acute episodes of illness, provided they have access to a range of life support, health, and mental health treatment and rehabilitation services." The plan focused on federal resources, notably those available under the Social Security Act. It asked for changes in SSI, SSDI, Medicare, Medicaid, and Social Services. The changes were designed to improve coverage for persons with mental illnesses and to eliminate disparities that impeded their integration into the community. The plan urged DHHS to adopt an incremental fiscal improvement strategy, to improve knowledge about this population and their needs, to develop a more effective workforce to assist them, and to improve collaboration with other federal departments that had important roles in influencing the availability of services and opportunities for this group.[62] The National Plan benefited from the invited contributions of service users, advocates, and national organizations, including the newly created National Alliance for the Mentally Ill (NAMI) representing the families of individuals with severe and persistent mental disorders.

The National Plan not only detailed the faults and shortcomings of the mental health system but offered a blueprint for future action. The plan, which originated in the deliberations of the PCMH, represented a watershed. Rather than existing in isolation, mental health had to be considered in relationship to the larger health care system and health policy. Many of the themes embodied in the abortive Mental Health Systems Act, recalled Tischler, "had an impact on how the government came to approach mental health services. . . . [including] federal–state partnerships, planning and accountability, and the integration of mental and other health services." Despite the political conservatism of the 1980s, a number of recommendations in the National Plan were implemented incrementally in the federal bureaucracy, thus lessening the impact of the Reagan administration's efforts to reduce the role of the federal government. The use of federal entitlement programs materially assisted persons with severe mental disorders and helped improve their lives. Nevertheless, care and treatment in the community for such individuals continued to pose challenges. In the community (and particularly in large urban areas) successful management depended on bringing together needed services administered by a variety of bureaucracies, each with its own culture, priorities, and preferred client populations. But only a small number of communities succeeded in integrating psychiatric care and treatment, social services, housing, and social support networks. The overwhelming majority of persons with severe and persistent mental illnesses continued to face a difficult future.

Less obvious but also important was the PCMH's stimulus to the development of a psychiatric epidemiology that, for better or worse, created a whole new set of issues. Daniel Freedman, an important figure in American psychiatry from the 1960s until his death in 1993, believed that the PCMH had created a "climate of informed concern" by focusing on the underserved and the need to bring "the mentally ill and disabled into undisputed full entitlement to professional and social services and gains from new knowledge." Its report had highlighted the need for a sound and useful knowledge base, which required a vigorous expansion of psychiatric epidemiology. "Diagnosis, prognosis and special social practices or behavioral and biomedical treatment," he insisted, "require the data that sophisticated epidemiology can create." Published in the prestigious *Archives of General Psychiatry,* his editorial was followed by two articles emphasizing the potential contributions of psychiatric epidemiology to administrators and policy makers. The discipline, according to Lee N. Robins, a major figure in the emergence of diagnostic psychiatry, "offers opportunities to explore questions about who gets ill and why, and to suggest methods for improving the mental health of the country." In subsequent years the discipline of psychiatric epidemiology grew rapidly and began to serve as an important tool to guide policy formulation and implementation.[63]

The history of the PCMH and the abortive legislation that followed illustrates the impact of social and political change on mental health policy. Between the 1940s and 1960s, a small number of strategically located individuals were able to reshape policy. But by the 1970s quite a different situation prevailed. The receptivity of the 1960s to innovation was followed by a decade of consolidation and retrenchment. Carter's fiscal conservatism constrained the PCMH's work. More important, the rise of groups that defined themselves in terms of race, gender, and ethnicity helped change the configuration of American politics. That such change benefited marginalized minorities, women, and persons with disabilities is clear. Admittedly, the demands for services by these new groups were not in any way intended to detract from the needs of persons with serious mental disorders. Nevertheless, the rise in consciousness of neglected social groups created demands for mental health services by those not mentally ill. At the same time the elevation of many behaviors to the status of pathological entities, perhaps best indicated by the publication of *DSM-III* in 1980 as well as by a dramatic increase in mental health personnel less concerned with serious mental disorders, contributed still more to the tendency to shift services away from individuals with more serious mental illnesses.[64]

The PCMH's experiences illuminate many of the difficulties that American society faces in dealing with health policy. Bureaucratic rivalries within and between governments; tensions and rivalries within the mental health professions; identity and interest-group politics; the difficulties of distinguishing the respective roles of elements such as poverty, racism, elitism, stigmatization, and unemployment in the etiology of mental disorders; and an illusory faith in the ability to prevent mental disorders all shaped the commission's deliberations. Its immediate impact on policy was minimal. The political conservatism that marked the presidencies of Ronald Reagan and George H. W. Bush precluded any decisive action during the 1980s. American society was not prepared to place a high priority on meeting the needs of persons whose serious mental illnesses created dependency. Yet the aftermath of the PCMH and the development of the National Plan inaugurated a serendipitous and incremental policy process that began to reshape mental health policy in subsequent years.

Chapter 5

From Legislative Repeal to Sequential Reform

The 1980s proved to be a decade of surprising success and increasing commitment to individuals with severe and persistent mental illnesses. To be sure, the Reagan administration was committed to policies that were designed to limit if not reduce the social welfare role of the federal government. The means chosen involved sharp reductions in taxation and the transfer of many social welfare responsibilities downward to state and local governments.[1] Although successful to some degree, these policies were mitigated by administrative actions taken by officials within the federal bureaucracy under the pressure of advocates and the Congress. Concerned that preoccupation with tax reduction and the shrinking or elimination of social programs might have devastating consequences for people with severe and persistent mental illnesses, the Congress passed new statutes that ensured that such individuals would have access to resources necessary to survive in the community. Thus the abortive effort to enact a program of broad comprehensive reform during the Carter administration was replaced instead by an emphasis on sequential incremental change that over time would help to improve the lives of people with serous mental disorders.

During the 1980s, following the disappointments over lost opportunities for more comprehensive reform during the previous decade, federal officials began to refocus on those who were most impaired.[2] Ironically, the unanticipated "quiet success" resulted from the piecemeal implementation of the recommendations of the National Plan for the Chronically Mentally Ill.[3] This success represented a shift from the radicalism of earlier broad reform proposals toward a more narrow but focused incrementalism.

The National Plan, however, added something new to incremental reform—a blueprint of specific recommendations suggesting a clear direction and a sequence of steps to achieve reform. The strategic choices of "sequentialism" replaced the opportunism of simple incrementalism.[4] In an era in which incremental reform was all that could be expected, sequentialism represented a more effective method of achieving reform goals. The National Plan set forth those objectives in specific recommendations to change both statutes and regulations governing important mainstream health and social welfare programs, including Medicare, Medicaid, and the disability programs of the Social Security Administration (SSA), which affected people with severe and persistent mental disorders. The emphasis was on specific recommendations that had all but disappeared from the recommendations of the PCMH and the provisions of the Mental Health Systems Act.

The narrowing focus on chronic mental illnesses and the push for incremental reform, however, was associated with a more fundamental redirection of social policy with respect to individuals with severe and persistent mental illnesses. Not only was there a shift to the most impaired, but there was also a broadening of the understanding of chronic mental illnesses.[5] A changing conceptual framework—community support—enlarged on the disease model of mental illnesses to encompass an expanded social welfare view of chronic mental illnesses that recognized the complex needs of individuals disabled by a mental disorder.[6] Within this framework the conceptualization of needs went beyond the need for traditional health, mental health, and substance abuse services to include housing, employment, education, vocational rehabilitation, and support services designed to promote full community integration. This novel approach ended the pattern of earlier policies that had been based on the belief that early treatment of mental illnesses would by themselves prevent chronicity and disability.[7] The optimism about prevention had been both idealistic and unsupported by evidence. The earlier faith in the efficacy of moral treatment, mental hygiene, and community mental health with its emphasis on deinstitutionalization raised hopes but ended up neglecting individuals with the most disabling conditions. The new approach emphasized social support and rehabilitation for individuals who already were disabled but who wished to be integrated into their communities.

Almost from its inception the CMHC program had been attacked for its disconnect from individuals with the most significant impairments, especially those in public mental hospitals.[8] The movement toward community mental health care and deinstitutionalization needed to be linked by services in the community that would meet the complex needs of the most impaired individuals who historically had been served by public hospitals. The concept of the community support system was developed to provide a strategic vision for the services that would meet those needs. It was accompanied by a broadened view of mental illnesses that conceptualized chronic mental illnesses as both a medical and a social welfare problem. In addition to specialized mental health services, a community support system was designed to provide housing, transportation, general medical and dental services, education and vocational rehabilitation, income and other social supports, and recognized and reinforced natural supports already in the community. Proponents referred to a community support system as a "network of caring and responsible people." [9]

The change in focus was especially evident in the new role of the NIMH, which was at the center of the development of the community support concept. In 1977 it created the Community Support Program (CSP) to promote its implementation. Even though the NIMH was responsible for the administration of the CMHC program, its Division of Mental Health Services Programs (which managed the CMHCs) began formulating the CSP in 1974 with a work group started by Lucy Ozarin and supported by NIMH director Bertram Brown and the Services Division director, Frank Ochberg, all of whom were psychiatrists. A task force was formed out of the original work group and was charged "to update the NIMH Hospital Improvement Program and the Hospital Staff Development Program." These two programs had been the only NIMH programs directed at assisting and improving the public mental hospital system, and the resources allocated to these programs were never substantial. The relative absence of support for public mental hospitals had been a sore point in many quarters, particularly among the National Association of State Mental Health Program Directors. The function of these two very small programs was about to be redirected toward community mental health but away from the CMHC program and toward the state mental health authorities.[10] Members of other NIMH divisions and several federal agencies were invited to the task force meetings, which were under the staff leadership of Judith Turner, William TenHoor, and G. Bart Stone. The CSP was officially launched as an NIMH program in 1977, and shortly thereafter, it began making grants to states to develop and implement community support systems. Steven S. Sharfstein, newly appointed director of the Division of Mental Health Services Programs, became chair of the CSP implementation group.[11]

The principles and content of the CSP were described in detail in an important 1978 paper by Turner and TenHoor in *Schizophrenia Bulletin,* a scientific journal published by the NIMH.[12] Appearing alongside articles on neurobiology and clinical trials of new treatments for schizophrenia, the publication in *Schizophrenia Bulletin* added legitimacy to the concept and the program. The stewards of CSP explained to their readers that serving individuals with severe mental disorders meant extending services beyond the boundaries of the traditional mental health services system. It meant more than hospitalization, medications, and psychotherapy. The new service system was designed to work in a partnership between the state mental health authority and some locus of responsibility at the local level with better lines of responsibility and accountability. Turner and TenHoor recognized a long-standing problem in mental health policy when they concluded that "perhaps the most critical factor contributing to inadequacies in community-based care is fragmentation and confusion of responsibility among the many federal, state, and local agencies whose programs have an impact on services to the mentally disabled in the community."[13] The recommendations went well beyond the CMHC approach to mental health services for individuals with severe and persistent mental disorders.

The CSP was encouraged by a confluence of forces and factors. The General Accounting Office 1977 study, *Returning the Mentally Disabled to the Community: Government Needs to Do More* provided the critical impetus to the CSP at the time of its initiation.[14] By 1978 nineteen states had been given $3.5 million in CSP grants. The resources went to the state mental health authorities, as had been the case for the hospital improvement programs from which CSP was born. States then let subcontracts to local programs to fund community support system implementation efforts. This tactic addressed prior concerns that the NIMH and its community programs (that is, the CMHCs) had largely ignored the state authorities. CSP explicitly linked the state to community services—and it proved to be an innovative approach to community mental health services. The program was boosted further by some of the recommendations of the PCMH and the provisions in the Mental Health Systems Act that looked to expand services for individuals with chronic mental illnesses. The latter had authorized the awarding of grants directly to the state mental health authorities, thus embodying a "new federalism" in mental health policy.[15]

When the Mental Health Systems Act was repealed almost entirely by the Omnibus Budget Reconciliation Act of 1981 in the first year of the Reagan administration, the CSP lost its chance for dramatic growth. Skillful and committed career staff members at NIMH, however, sustained the program in spite of administration threats to its existence. The Omnibus Budget Reconciliation Act replaced targeted federal service grants to organizations such as CMHCs in favor of a block grant, effectively ending the federal CMHC programs. Although the block grant went directly to states, they used it to further the agenda of the CSP. Further, Public Law 99-660 called for all states to develop a plan for the care of individuals with severe mental illnesses, based on the CSP model. In this way the basic constructs of the community support reform were advanced in small steps, in spite of the repeal of the Mental Health Systems Act.[16]

In fact the most enduring support for CSP came from the National Plan, whose recommendations were designed to facilitate the implementation of community support programs using mainstream resources in tandem with traditional state categorical mental health dollars. CSP was a bold new approach to services designed to address the historic problem of policy fragmentation. The plan provided a blueprint for advancing this reform. The enthusiasm surrounding CSP and the presence of a roadmap of recommended incremental changes in the National Plan meant that the demise of the Mental Health Systems Act would not end mental health reform.

Nowhere was the power of the federal bureaucracy to shape policy by administrative actions better illustrated than in the effort by Reagan officials to remove individuals from the disability rolls. Between March 1981 and June 1983 hundreds of thousands of disabled individuals were purged from the SSA disability rolls as a result of an accelerated process of "Continuing Disability Investigations."[17] The purge was motivated by a desire to save government resources by removing as many as half a million people who were thought to no longer qualify for their disability benefits. The process singled out younger beneficiaries who were disproportionately entitled to benefits on the basis of a mental impairment. This travesty of social policy eventually was rectified as the first of many sequential steps implementing the National Plan, an agenda for action that had been developed as a government response to the PCMH. Reversing the process of disability investigations began a decade of stepwise reform guided by the blueprint offered in the National Plan.[18]

The disability investigation process began as an apparent effort in good government by the newly elected Reagan administration. Beginning with the transition between administrations, the Office of Management and Budget (OMB) began to look for places to save substantial resources in order to fulfill President Reagan's promise in his first congressional budget message to cut

$48.6 billion in federal expenditures. The SSDI program gave them an opportunity to save as much as $3.45 billion over the next five years.[19] Budget cutters seized on the chance to implement provisions of the Social Security Amendments of 1980, passed in June of the final year of the Carter administration. These amendments mandated "periodic reviews" of all SSDI beneficiaries who were not considered "permanently disabled" to determine continuing eligibility. The law called for the reviews to occur once every three years, beginning in January 1982. President Reagan's OMB required the SSA to begin the process in March 1981, just weeks after the inauguration and without any chance for advanced preparation by the SSA.[20]

The 1980 legislation had been a response to the dramatic expansion of the SSDI rolls during the early 1970s. Between 1970 and 1975 the number of disabled worker beneficiaries grew by 45 percent to 2.6 million in 1976, costing $10 billion annually.[21] By the time of the legislation, however, SSDI program growth had already begun to decline, according to SSA's own studies.[22] In 1980 new awards had fallen from a high in 1975 of 592,000 to 390,000, the lowest level in a decade.[23] During the Reagan transition, GAO staff stationed in SSA's Baltimore headquarters made known to the new administration their rough estimates that about 20 percent of individuals on SSDI did not meet the criteria for continued eligibility. The GAO staff members did not, however, make known their reservations about their estimates or share their concerns about the feasibility of an accelerated process of disability investigations. They rather appeared to be currying favor with the new administration.[24]

In March 1981 all hell broke loose. The accelerated schedule of disability investigations began, and within months the abrupt termination of SSDI benefits captured the attention of advocates and the Congress alike. Horror stories emerged of SSDI beneficiaries committing suicide in despondency over their loss of disability payments. Terminations reached their highest level ever in the last quarter of 1981 as 50 percent of all disability investigations resulted in a cessation of benefits. Advocates for individuals with mental disorders were particularly aroused, because younger SSDI beneficiaries were disproportionately represented among those who were subject to review—they were not considered permanently disabled—and individuals with mental disorders constituted a large proportion of these younger beneficiaries. The problem worsened in January 1982, when the SSI program was added to the accelerated process of investigations.[25] The SSI rolls were even more heavily populated by younger individuals with mental impairments who had never worked enough to earn SSDI coverage. Their benefits were meager to begin with, and now they were forced to fend without income supports, without the Medicaid coverage that usually accompanied their SSI eligibility, and without the skills to find work. The rhetoric reached a heated pitch by late 1982, leading Congressman Claude Pepper to accuse the administration of "cruel and callous policies designed to strike terror into the hearts of crippled people all across America."[26]

Disability and mental health advocates were outraged by the terminations.[27] Even among government officials there was growing doubt that the terminations were justified. By 1982, SSA policy leaders and senior administration officials admitted privately that they had doubts about the wisdom of their plan. Moreover, they realized that they had created a domestic policy problem that was embarrassing the White House. Publicly, however, they testified that they were just implementing the 1980 Social Security Amendments, guided by the GAO report on eligibility. Paul Simmons, chief of policy for SSA, and Associate Commissioner for Disability John Svahn explained that the standard for disability was very strict.[28] To qualify for benefits individuals had to demonstrate that they were unable to perform any "substantial gainful activity" that existed in the national economy. That meant either "meeting or equaling" one of the Listings of Mental Impairment, a set of medical criteria operationalizing disability, or being found to have too little "residual functional capacity" based on limitations, age, and work experience to be able to maintain competitive employment. Furthermore, the burden of proof was on the claimant to demonstrate disabled status as a result of a "medically determinable physical or mental impairment."

In retrospect it is clear that the SSA and GAO exaggerated the estimates of the number of individuals who were no longer disabled and thus inappropriately receiving benefits.[29] It is also clear that moving up the date for starting the disability investigations and accelerating the process undermined the good-government intent of the reviews. The process was too aggressive, too fast, and implemented without adequate planning. Adding SSI to the original plan for SSDI reviews merely exacerbated the problem, since it purged the rolls of indigent individuals who lacked work experience and had little prospect for recovery or self-sufficiency. What also became clear was that SSA was not following its own procedures for adjudicating claims of disability, thus providing advocates the opportunity to seek a remedy in the courts.[30]

The fundamental claim in the court cases that followed rested on the expectation that every SSA disability claimant was entitled to an individualized assessment of the capacity to work, once it was determined that the individual's impairment exceeded a threshold test of severity. In 1981 and 1982 a series of lawsuits were filed by lawyers on behalf of individuals whose disability benefits were "ceased"—to use the terminology of the disability investigation process. A class action suit filed in Utah in 1982, *H.J. v. Schweiker,* was the first systemic challenge, but it could allege only that SSA actions "bear no factual or rational relationship to the actual psychiatric condition and disability of the plaintiffs involved."[31] The court denied the motion for a preliminary injunction because there was no evidence demonstrating a systematic violation of plaintiffs' rights. The next case was based on better evidence. In 1982 plaintiffs' lawyers in *Mental Health Association of Minnesota (MHAM) v. Schweiker* discovered internal SSA documents that suggested that individuals in the disability investigation process had been denied the individualized assessment to which they were entitled. Specifically, their cases were reviewed on the basis of the Listings of Impairment but not on residual functional capacity. Individuals were denied benefits if they could not meet the Listings and, as a result, were considered able to perform any work in the national economy. Plaintiffs sought an injunction against the review process as well as a redetermination of their cases. In December 1982 the court found in favor of the plaintiffs, but the judgment and the injunction applied only in the six states in SSA's Chicago region with federal court jurisdiction.[32] A class action case in another region attracted the attention and support of the state of New York and New York City, which decided to join in the suit against the federal government in February 1983 *(City of New York v. Heckler).* Once again the court found for the plaintiffs, and both *MHAM* and *City of New York* prevailed on appeal, demonstrating that SSA's process violated its own procedures. Judge Jack Weinstein was outraged that SSA had operated under a "clandestine" policy, which "pressured" physicians to make hasty and unsubstantiated determinations, demonstrating a "supremacy of bureaucracy over professional medical judgments."[33] The Supreme Court sustained these cases in 1986 with a unanimous decision in *Bowen v. City of New York.* This ended the complex legal proceedings with SSA and paved the way for a redetermination of the cases of every individual whose benefits had been terminated in the disability investigation process of the prior years.[34]

SSA policy on determinations of disability due to mental disorder had strayed from its own regulatory definition of disability to an idiosyncratic definition based in its unpublished program operations manual system. Late in 1982 the GAO determined that according to the manual, there was a "virtual presumption" that an individual who did not meet the Listings retained the residual functional capacity to perform unskilled work. The drive to render the assessment of mental impairment more objective had led to a policy of ignoring the influence of "vocational factors" such as age, education, and prior work experience on functional capacity for competitive employment. Instead, SSA focused almost entirely on the signs and symptoms of mental disorders. The reliance on the unpublished criteria rather than on regulations meant that policies were not exposed to public comment and criticism, which created an "adjudicative climate" that shaped decisions that were out of touch with professional judgment and with SSA's own regulations.[35]

While the SSA and the Reagan administration fought the class action lawsuits and appealed the decisions to successively higher courts, they also recognized the political liabilities that they had incurred. Consequently, they began a process designed to correct their errors. The policy reversal began in June 1983 when Secretary of Health and Human Services Margaret Heckler, who had been SSA commissioner during the disability investigation period, called for a moratorium on the review process. Heckler exempted from the eligibility redeterminations two-thirds of the beneficiaries with mental impairments to avoid "hardships and heartbreaks." The "Continuing Disability Investigation" process was relabeled a "Continuing Disability Review" process. The policy shift represented recognition of the harshness and aggressiveness of the term describing the government's efforts to save resources by "investigating" and terminating the benefits of disabled individuals.[36]

By 1983, SSA recognized that it had serious problems with its disability determination process. SSA realized that it needed to revise the Listings of Mental Impairments, which were the regulations that identified and listed the mental impairments that qualfied a claimant for disability payments. The Listings that were current at that time listed only a few large categories of mental disorders (for example, organic brain syndromes, psychoses, and neuroses) and the symptoms (for example, disorientation, hallucinations, and anxiety) and functional limitations (for example, poor concentration) associated with them. Legal discovery in the court cases revealed that SSA had overemphasized symptoms of impairment as a proxy for functional limitations, when research indicated that there was not as strong a correlation as the Listings of Mental Impairment implied. Furthermore, the Listings did not use current diagnostic criteria for establishing the presence of a medically determinable impairment and had a very high threshold for the functional limitations that operationalized disability. The Residual Functional Capacity measures were also judged inadequate by mental health experts who testified at the trials, and the evidence indicated that such determinations were not being conducted in the review process.

Early in 1983 SSA convened a work group, co-sponsored and co-chaired by the APA. The APA had been among the most visible critics of the SSA, and some of its experts had testified in the court cases.[37] Included in the work group were representatives of the other disciplinary organizations for psychologists, nurses, and social workers, as well as representatives of the Mental Health Law Project (now the Bazelon Center for Mental Health Law), which had been the successful litigant in the lawsuits. Representing the government were individuals from the SSA's central office in Baltimore, members of its medical and policy staff, as well as representatives of several State Disability Determination Services and other government agencies, including the NIMH and the Health Care Financing Administration.[38] The work group was charged with revising the Listings of Mental Impairment and the Residual Functional Capacity measures and making recommendations to improve the reliability and validity of the process of disability determination for adults and, later, for children.

The work group process began with defensiveness on the part of the staff of SSA, followed by further criticism of SSA from virtually all of the participants. SSA finally came to the realization that it would be necessary to change its policies. The work group proposed relatively conservative changes to the existing regulations, in order to increase their acceptability to higher-ups in the Reagan administration and also because the regulations themselves were not the whole problem. The "adjudicative climate" needed to be altered to resume the orderly and legal process of disability determination that did not automatically presume that those individuals who did not meet an outdated set of Listings of Mental Impairment could perform unskilled work.

The new Listings were designed to correct the policy and to create a new climate that followed regulatory policy and resumed determinations of residual functional capacity.[39] The new Listings built upon the old Listings, adopting the same basic approach. Both the new and the old regulations identified a set of signs and symptoms of specific categories of mental disorder, a set of "A criteria" identifying the impairments that a claimant should demonstrate and document as evidence of a "medically determinable mental disorder." The "A criteria" were associated with a set of "B criteria" that characterized the types of functional limitations indicative of disability due to the signs and symptoms of the mental impairments identified in the "A criteria" of the Listings. The functional limitations included activities of daily living (such as maintaining personal hygiene and other aspects of caring for oneself), social interaction, concentration, and adaptive functioning (such as the ability to deal with stressful situations without an exacerbation of symptoms).

The "B criteria" were the same for all of the categories of impairment, except for mental retardation, which defined disability according to the IQ level. The old Listings defined the threshold of disability for four categories of mental impairment as marked functional limitation in all four areas of the "B criteria." In the "adjudicative climate" of the Continuing Disability Investigation process individuals assessed as able to perform any of the wide array of functions described in the "B" criteria were not disabled according to the Listings. If they were not disabled by the Listings in this climate, they also were not assessed for residual capacity, and were found to be not disabled.

The new Listings increased the number of categories of impairment from four to eight and used "A criteria" derived from the newly published APA's *DSM-III*. These "A criteria" were more reliable indicators of the presence of a mental impairment than the old "A criteria" and were more widely recognized by mental health practitioners. For example, the "A criteria" for affective disorders included all of the *DSM-III* criteria for major depression, such as sleep and appetite disturbance. In the old Listings substance abuse was considered to be a potentially disabling condition by SSA regulations, but there was no specific Listing for this category of mental impairment. Instead, an individual might qualify on the basis of substance abuse by "reference" to another category of impairment, such as "organic mental disorder" or "liver disease," for example. The work group recommended a set of "A criteria" specific to each category of impairment, including substance abuse.

The work group proposed changes in the threshold on the "B criteria" for a determination of disability, so that only two or three of the four categories of functional limitations needed to be markedly restricted for a determination of disability. Initially the work group proposed that the threshold of Listing-level disability should be "marked limitation" in two of the four "B criteria," where "marked" was defined on a ordinal scale as "more than moderate but less than extreme limitation." Many hours were spent trying to achieve agreement on this less-than-perfect definition. The lawyers in the work group noted that this standard was not so different from the standards of evidence used in legal matters, ranging from "preponderance" through "clear and convincing" to "beyond a reasonable doubt."

The lack of precision in this definition, coupled with the addition of new categories of impairment with which SSA had little experience, led some members of the work group, particularly those with SSA and its state agencies, to make a counterproposal to setting the threshold at two areas of marked limitation. They suggested raising the standard to three areas of marked functional limitation for some of the categories of impairments that were less likely to be disabling (such as anxiety, substance abuse, and somatoform disorders). The proposal remained at two areas of marked limitation for affective disorders (such as depression and bipolar disorder) and for schizophrenia and dementia, delirium and amnestic disorders (previously referred to as "organic brain syndromes"). Some work group members felt that the level should be three for all categories, noting that it had been four in the old Listings, but advocates for setting a lower standard argued that it should be two for all categories. The initial compromise prevailed, and the proposal was set at two marked limitations for the conditions that were more likely on average to be severely disabling and three for the others that were considered less likely to be disabling.

In addition, the work group proposed a new "C criterion" for schizophrenia and related psychotic disorders which considered treatment, supports, and accommodating living arrangement that permitted individuals to function reasonably well, in spite of the persistence of limitations that would emerge when the individual left such protected settings and arrangements. The new regulations proposed that an individual could be found disabled if the "A criteria" for schizophrenia were met and the individual had been living for two years in a supportive situation that rendered him or her less symptomatic but still disabled, with a return of functional limitations that would meet the "B criteria" if the individual were outside the supportive arrangement.

Once the work group arrived at its proposal, the draft regulation was prepared by SSA staff and made its way through the process of rule making. The first step involved a formal "Notice of Proposed Rule Making" that would be released in the *Federal Register* for public comment.[40] Prior to public release there were many internal deliberations within the Department of Health and Human Services and within the OMB about the proposed regulations. Substance abuse was dropped as a category of impairment; this proposal was considered too controversial. OMB initially proposed setting the "B criteria" for all impairments at three areas of marked limitation, and officials were wary of the "C criterion." Internal advocates prevailed in sustaining the views of the work group on both issues, and the Notice of Proposed Rule Making was released more or less as the work group had recommended. Comments sustained the proposed rules, and the Final Rule was almost identical to the initial recommendation.

While the work group was meeting in 1983 and 1984, Congress developed legislation to correct the disability determination process and related matters of SSA policy. Although they were aware of SSA's internal efforts to redress the policy problems, members of Congress, led by Representative J. J. Pickle (D-Texas) and Senator John Heinz (R-Pennsylvania), were adamant that legislation was required to hold SSA's feet to the fire. The result was a series of regulatory changes in the Listings and in Residual Functional Capacity measures, as well as the passage of the Disability Reform Act of 1984 (PL 98-460).[41] The new law placed a moratorium on all disability reviews involving mental impairments until the Listings could be revised. SSA was required to identify and reassess all of the individuals who, since March 1981, had had their benefits terminated for disability due to mental impairment, and who had appealed their termination as of June 7, 1983. Individuals whose terminations were reversed were entitled to collect back-benefits. Those individuals whose terminations were not on appeal could reapply and have their claim adjudicated under the new criteria, and, if found disabled, they too would receive back-benefits. A new "medical improvement standard" for terminating benefits was implemented for all disability reviews that stipulated that beneficiaries could not be deprived of benefits as "able to work" unless their underlying impairment had improved medically. No longer could individuals lose their benefits on the basis of an assessment of a change in functional capacity and a determination that they were no longer disabled, unless there was also a finding of "medical improvement."

The Disability Reform Act also required SSA to change many of its procedures. A psychiatrist or psychologist had to complete the medical portion of the case review for all claimants alleging disability on the basis of mental impairment, before benefits could be denied. Special efforts were required for all mental impairment claims to improve the collection of medical evidence, especially from physicians who had been treating the claimant. Adjudicators were directed to give additional weight to the judgments of these so-called treating sources. Finally, SSA was required to report to the Congress on studies it fielded related to work and work evaluations.

The initial impact of the disability legislation was almost immediate. SSA's new mental impairment standards became effective in 1985. Many of the other provisions were slower to be implemented, but the act set a new legislative mandate for reform of SSA's disability programs and management of individuals with mental impairments.

Some members of the work group and other advocates lobbying the Congress on the Disability Reform Act had been participants in the preparation of the National Plan, and many others were aware of its recommendations dealing with the SSA disability program. In fact, the National Plan had one general recommendation to improve the disability determination process and six specific SSA-related recommendations.[42]

The most important recommendation of the National Plan for the SSA disability programs was to change the criteria for determining disability. With respect to SSDI and SSI this problem was addressed in the wake of the disability investigations policy nightmare. By the mid-1980s the new Listings of Mental Impairment and Residual Function Capacity assessment process were in place. An APA study sponsored by SSA demonstrated that these new tools were reliable and valid, particularly when adequate information was available for a claimant. The rate of "allowances" (that is, the proportion of claimants who were granted or "allowed" benefits) rose from 38.8 percent in FY 1983 to 52.3 percent in FY 1986.[43]

With respect to SSDI the National Plan had also recommended the elimination of the "substantial gainful activity" test for individuals who returned to work.[44] This recommendation was an effort to extend to SSDI beneficiaries some of the incentives to return to work that were already part of the SSI return-to-work program. The National Plan expressed concern about the difficulty of getting benefits when disabled and the disincentives for beneficiaries' returning to work when a precipitous loss of benefits would result. The recommendation to drop the gainful activity test still had not been implemented in 1991 according to an analysis that followed up on the recommendations of the National Plan a decade later.[45]

For SSI the National Plan had made four specific recommendations in addition to the general recommendation about disability criteria. The plan had called for improvements in the program that assisted individuals who were being discharged from state mental hospitals in obtaining benefits that were needed to provide income for community living. Some problems remained, but this recommendation was essentially achieved by the time of the ten-year follow-up to the National Plan. The same was true for the three other recommendations that called for incremental improvements to the Section 1619 work-incentive program.

There were additional nonspecific National Plan recommendations for the SSA disability program that related to linking disability benefits to health care benefits. The link was vital to ensure that individuals with disabling impairments would be able to obtain health care and possibly move toward recovery and return to work. The incentives in the programs, however, often made the recovery process more difficult. For example, SSDI beneficiaries were required to wait for two years once on disability benefits before becoming eligible for

Medicare, and at the time of the National Plan twelve states did not extend Medicaid benefits to SSI recipients. In a series of sequential steps, proceeding from the tragedy of the disability investigation process, by 1991 all but one of the specific National Plan recommendations for the SSA disability programs had been implemented. Advocates aware of those recommendations had pushed for reforms. The same was true for the National Plan recommendations for Medicare and Medicaid, the financing programs of the federal government that were linked to disability. These health care financing programs began to take on special importance for providing mental health services to the most impaired individuals with mental disorders.

In 1980 the framers of the National Plan had also recognized the great potential of Medicaid for financing the public mental health service system that had traditionally been financed by categorical grants from state mental health authorities.[46] In 1971 mental health services accounted for about 11.9 percent of the total Medicaid budget—or approximately $1.6 billion. By 1987 this amount rose to $16.7 billion (including services for substance abuse)—or about 20 percent of the Medicaid total.[47] The designers of the National Plan had set in motion a series of changes that resulted in Medicaid's becoming the dominant funder of mental health services. They appreciated that the state–federal financing partnership that provided health care coverage for individuals who were poor (qualifying for Aid to Families with Dependent Children [AFDC]) or aged and disabled (qualifying for SSI) could become a source of fuel for the engine of increasing demand for mental health services in community settings.

The keys to the incremental success achieved by mental health advocates on behalf of Medicaid and Medicare reform were major amendments to entitlement legislation and the budget reconciliation process that had become the major avenue for federal legislation.[48] During the Reagan years and into the first Bush administration, most federal legislation in health and social welfare fell into a single annual budget bill, known as the "budget reconciliation." Since the 1981 Omnibus Budget Reconciliation Act that had repealed the Mental Health Systems Act and replaced it with block grants, the advocates learned that if they wanted to push for legislative reform, they had to get their proposals into the annual budget reconciliation bill. The benefit of this strategy was the enormity and the complexity of the process, making it possible to bury a small legislative proposal in the larger bill without attracting adverse attention from the budgeteers. The same legislative process that had dashed the hopes of the reformers behind the Mental Health Systems Act in 1981 became the favored tactic of the advocates for the rest of the decade. The Comprehensive Omnibus Budget Reconciliation Acts (OBRAs and COBRAs) of each succeeding year contained small provisions of mental health reform affecting Medicaid and Medicare that would shape mental health services policy for a quarter of a century.

The deinstitutionalization and community care movements resulted in individuals with severe and persistent mental disorders living in community settings and using community-based services. The federally funded community mental health centers were neither prepared for nor interested in dealing with such individuals, and states had quite limited resources.[49] The Medicaid partnership with the federal government meant that state dollars appropriated for mental health services could draw down federal Medicaid dollars in a match that varied from state to state from one-for-one (50 percent match in most states) to a match rate of 78 percent in some poorer states. The designers of Medicaid, however, had imposed a number of limitations on mental health services within the 1965 design of the program.[50] The National Plan identified these limitations and recommended a series of changes to improve the financing of mental health services for individuals with severe and persistent mental disorders who qualified for Medicaid.

Title XIX of the Social Security Act requires every state Medicaid program to offer a set of basic services, including physician services; outpatient hospital services; early periodic screening, diagnosis, and treatment (EPSDT) services for children; and inpatient hospital and nursing home services. The inpatient and nursing home benefits excluded care in "institutions for mental disease" for individuals between the ages of twenty-two and sixty-four years. Institutions for mental disease were defined as facilities that provided primarily psychiatric treatment and where half of the residents had a diagnosis of a mental disorder. Freestanding public and private psychiatric hospitals were considered in the same category, as were nursing homes that specialized in psychiatric care.

Medicaid also permitted states to pay for optional services, including care in institutions for mental diseases, for individuals twenty-one years and younger and aged sixty-five years and older; prescription drugs; clinic services (called the "clinic option"); and other medical and rehabilitation services provided by licensed professionals. Within these federal guidelines states defined the precise benefits, including placing more limitations on mental health services than on general medical services. The National Plan found that additional limits often were imposed on outpatient visits and inpatient length of stay for mental health services. It concluded that there was "an obvious bias against psychiatry." States also had an option to expand eligibility beyond AFDC and SSI beneficiaries to those deemed "Medically Needy" who had high medical expenses. At the time of the National Plan not all individuals receiving AFDC or SSI benefits qualified for Medicaid. In particular, twelve states used Section 209(b) to restrict the eligibility criteria for Medicaid, requiring stricter definitions of disability or indigence.[51]

The National Plan made thirteen Medicaid recommendations that fell into three categories: expanding community services, modifying the institutions for mental diseases rule, and improving the link between Medicaid and SSI.[52] The plan developers considered changes in Medicaid the highest priority. Although only five of the thirteen recommendations had been adopted by 1991, they changed the face of community mental health services in profound ways.[53]

The National Plan also advanced seven recommendations to expand community mental health services.[54] Recommendations to evaluate state Medicaid plans for evidence of discrimination and to analyze state decision making that might reward inappropriate services were not adopted. Perhaps these broad recommendations to overhaul Medicaid mental health policy, recommendations implying discrimination and inappropriate reimbursements, were too challenging for action in the incremental and conservative climate of the 1980s. Whatever the reason, they were not implemented.[55] Advocates were successful, however, in convincing the Congress to initiate a targeted case management option, to encourage the states and their Medicaid programs to expand psychosocial rehabilitation services, and to permit reimbursement of mental health clinics under the broad clinic option. In addition, advocates achieved partial implementation of the recommendation to provide states with technical assistance to promote innovations in the use of Medicaid to finance mental health services. The NIMH and private foundations offered resources to help independent organizations (for example, the National Conference of State Legislatures, the National Association of State Mental Health Program Directors, and the National Mental Health Association) to provide limited technical assistance.[56]

The targeted case management option was the most important of these changes, since it was central to implementing community support services in each community. Also called "resource management," this service was provided by an individual "case manager," someone who guided an individual experiencing a severe mental illness through the complex service system. The case manager was supposed to assist individuals in obtaining needed resources and treatment, linking them with myriad direct services and benefits. The targeted case management benefit was implemented in a series of sequential steps.[57] First, COBRA 1985 (PL 99-272) gave states the option of providing these services for an indefinite period, so long as the case management services did not duplicate another service and were not themselves therapeutic services. States could target the services on the basis of a variety of factors, including geographic region, clinical condition, or age. Second, COBRA 1986 (PL 99-509) specifically permitted targeting of case management to individuals with "chronic mental illness." Third, the Budget Reconciliation Act of 1987 (PL 100-203) amended the law further to restrict case management payments only to providers "capable of ensuring that the individuals receive needed services." This meant that case managers had to be connected to the public mental health system providing the services to meet client needs.

The Omnibus Reconciliation Act of 1990 (PL 101-508) provided a statutory basis for improving psychosocial rehabilitation services. Several states had improved Medicaid benefits for these services on their own during the 1980s, following the recommendations of the National Plan. The ability to provide rehabilitation services "off-site" (such as in a client's home or in a homeless shelter) as well as "on-site" (such as in a service program) was a major feature of this benefit. The 1990 legislation made it explicit that psychosocial rehabilitation services could be provided "off-site." This opened up the benefit to pay for some of the critical components of a community support system, including assertive community treatment—an important evidence-based service for some of the most disabled clients of the mental health service system.

No legislation was needed to apply the clinic option to mental health services. States chose to implement this recommendation, following the lead of the recommendations in the National Plan regarding the expansion of mental health services. This policy change used the federal Medicaid match to add resources to the ability of the public mental health system to respond to the demand for community mental health services by deinstitutionalized clients of the mental health system living in the community. Advocates for this and other Medicaid policy reforms were guided by the National Plan.

Advocates were less successful in getting a respite care benefit option adopted, in spite of support from Senator John Chafee (R-Rhode Island).[58] This recommendation called for Medicaid to pay for brief periods of residential care for individuals who were living in stable condition outside of residential settings with live-in caregivers—to give the caregivers a brief respite from their essential care-giving responsibility. Medicaid did not adopt this recommendation, nor did it accept any of the National Plan recommendations related to improved payments for 24-hour care.

The sole recommendation of the National Plan related to 24-hour care and institutions for mental diseases that *was* enacted established standards for nursing homes as a part of national nursing home reform. States had responded to the "institution for mental diseases" rule by transferring patients from state mental hospitals, where Medicaid could not be used to finance care for residents aged twenty-two to sixty-four, to nursing homes that did not qualify as institutions for mental diseases but whose residents could receive Medicaid federal financial resources. Many considered this policy of "transinstitutionalization" to be undesirable, since general nursing homes that did not qualify as mental institutions by definition probably were not skilled in caring for individuals with severe and persistent mental disorders. The National Plan had identified the huge population of individuals in nursing homes in the late 1970s and recommended care in alternative community settings that would be better able to meet the needs of residents with disabling mental illnesses.

For the first five or six years following the National Plan there was little policy activity related to improving care in nursing homes. In 1986, however, the Institute of Medicine issued a report critical of the quality of care in nursing homes and recommended policy changes.[59] The ensuing policy debate included the issue of mental illnesses that the institute report had neglected. The Omnibus Budget Reconciliation Act of 1987 (Subtitle C of PL 100-203) had the following provisions for individuals with a mental disorder diagnosis:

- Individuals with a mental disorder other than dementia could not be admitted unless they required this level of care and did not otherwise require "active treatment" that ordinarily would require a hospital level of care.
- Residents needed to undergo a similar assessment for ongoing stay.
- Individuals who had been resident for less than 30 days and did not need this level of care must be discharged.
- Plans of care must be developed to meet the needs for care, including psychosocial needs, determined in a comprehensive assessment of all residents.
- Nursing homes were required to provide these needed services.
- The rights of residents were to be protected from a range of abuses, including seclusion and physical and chemical restraint (that is, use

of psychoactive medications) used for convenience of the staff or as punishment for behavioral disturbance.

• Residents who did not meet the requirements for continued stay and were scheduled for discharge must have community placements described by the state in Alternative Disposition Plans.

Technical amendments in the budget act of 1990 dealt with some controversial elements of pre-admission screening and some of the problems that had led to a delay in implementation of nursing home reform. The law made it clear that nursing homes were expected to provide the care needed by residents and that Medicaid must pay for the services. The so-called Pre-admission Screening and Resident Review caused much consternation and ultimately affected comparatively few individuals. Its direct beneficial impact was small, although it represented an important acknowledgment of the role of mental health services in nursing homes and problems in financing appropriate services.

Not all of the advocates and their organizations supported the National Plan recommendations related to expansion of institutions for mental diseases.[60] Many feared that such policy changes would reverse the trend toward community care and increase the use of hospital and other residential and nursing home services. Without strong and consistent advocacy, the plan recommendations for a demonstration to test a service model for an intermediate care center for mental health and to develop special mental illness care standards for intermediate care facilities for mental retardation were not adopted. These issues were partly addressed when the Catastrophic Health Insurance Act of 1988 (PL 100-360) permitted Medicaid payments to intermediate care facilities with fewer than sixteen residents regardless of diagnosis. This service model was losing favor by the late 1980s, however, as mental health service innovators championed "supported housing," serving individuals in their own homes or apartments with clinical and social support. These changes rendered the plan recommendations inappropriate by 1991.

There was only one other change in policy affecting nursing homes, and it was a minor clarification in the definition of an institution for mental diseases. At the urging of NIMH, Medicaid agreed to clarify the definition of the so-called 50 percent rule for residents in nursing homes. Residents with a primary diagnosis of Alzheimer's disease or a related dementia would no longer be counted in the determination of whether the resident population of the facility exceeded 50 percent of residents with a mental disorder diagnosis. As most of the residents who were at risk of being counted against the 50 percent ceiling had a dementia diagnosis, this rule change prevented many nursing homes from being labeled as a mental institution and thus ineligible for Medicaid payments. The rule change was also implemented with the expectation that it would increase the likelihood that individuals with mental disorders and the behavioral complications of dementia would receive appropriate services without losing Medicaid financing. Thomas Hoyer, a Health Care Financing Administration official, championed this small reform within his agency.[61]

The recommendation to amend the definition of an institution for mental diseases to exclude private, freestanding hospitals was unsuccessful. Medicaid was not inclined to treat facility types differently on the basis of auspices, as there was no apparent clinical difference between freestanding hospitals. As noted above, strong advocates for community-based services also were divided about any recommendation to increase financing for hospital services. The several recommendations of the National Plan relating to mental institutions and other forms of 24-hour care were controversial and would have been expensive in a time of fiscal conservatism.

Neither of the National Plan's recommendations to expand SSI-based eligibility for Medicaid broadly—and to make some individuals with a mental disorder "presumptively disabled" and thus qualified for Medicaid—was enacted. Over time the states on their own expanded the "Medically Needy" option to cover more individuals who were disabled by a mental disorder, but no broad Medicaid-sponsored effort to expand the number of enrollees was in place a decade after the National Plan was released in 1980. Improvements in SSA rules on mental impairment, however, did expand Title XIX eligibility. SSI eligibility increased dramatically during the 1980s in part due to the reforms described in the previous section.[62]

The National Plan targeted Medicaid for its most ambitious recommendations. It recognized the role that Medicaid could play in expanding mental health services for individuals with severe and persistent mental illnesses. Medicaid also provided coverage for individuals with more acute mental health problems, eligible through AFDC. As a result, Medicaid would become the dominant payer for mental health services over the next decade. The developers of the National Plan had not imagined as important a role for Medicare. Modeled on private insurance with a more medical model of coverage, Medicare did not figure prominently in the National Plan—but the sequence of changes that were to occur in Medicare's mental health benefit were to set precedents for improved mental health coverage more broadly.

When Medicare legislation was passed as Title XVIII of the Social Security Act in 1965, it provided insurance coverage for aged and disabled (SSDI) beneficiaries for mental health as well as general health services.[63] Coverage for mental health services, however, was more limited than for general health services in a pattern of underinsurance that was typical of private health insurance of the day. The hospital insurance portion (Part A) limited coverage to 190 days in a lifetime for care in a freestanding public or private hospital, while care in a general hospital for treatment of mental disorders was covered on the same basis as for other conditions. The voluntary coverage for supplemental medical insurance (Part B) limited outpatient treatment for "nervous and mental disease" to $500 of service per year with a co-payment rate of 50 percent.[64] This effectively limited Medicare's obligation to $250 in payments for outpatient mental health care. In addition, Medicare paid for little in the way of related services, particularly not the array of psychosocial and supportive services needed for individuals with severe mental disorders, which were covered under Medicaid.

The benefit limitations in Medicare were typical of private insurance coverage for mental health services, which were designed to restrict costs. There was widespread concern that providing insurance coverage for treating mental disorders would be too expensive.[65] Insurers called this concern "moral hazard," that the price-lowering effect of insurance would stimulate demand. In fact, early efforts at private insurance coverage had led to increases in expenditures. The strict limits ($250 annual maximum) and higher co-payments (50 percent versus 20 percent for general health services) were imposed on mental health services to control this level of spending, espcially for psychotherapy. Congress felt that other mental health services, particularly long-term treatment in freestanding psychiatric hospitals, were the financial responsibility of the states and should not be shifted to the federal government through Medicare. These policy rationales had been used, along with skepticism about the effectiveness of mental health treatments, to block efforts to achieve "parity" (that is, nondiscriminatory, equivalent) coverage of mental health services in private insurance as well as in Medicare.

The drive for parity among mental health advocates preceded the National Plan. President Kennedy had directed the Civil Service Commission to cover mental health services on the same basis as general medical services in health insurance for federal employees.[66] Federal employees enjoyed parity for a decade before cost increases reversed the policy and mental health benefits eroded. There also were discussions of parity during the Nixon years, when national health insurance was under consideration, and again during the Carter

Commission. Parity for Medicare was a special case, because it required a statutory change, as the outpatient limits were embedded in Title XVIII of the Social Security Act itself. This made the change more difficult to achieve. So in 1980 the National Plan made a single, modest recommendation regarding Medicare: increase the annual limit to $750 (from $250) and reduce the co-payment rate to 20 percent. The plan did, however, discuss the additional barriers to care, discussed above, as well as the two-year wait for Medicare for SSDI beneficiaries.[67]

In the first few years after the National Plan, a Medicare policy issue that had not been anticipated by the Plan was the first to affect the mental health community. Ironically, it was not an issue of parity but rather a desire to remain outside of the usual Medicare payment system for inpatient care that activated the mental health policy world in the early 1980s.

In 1982 Congress passed the Tax Equity and Fiscal Responsibility Act (PL 97-248), which placed cost controls on Medicare payments for all inpatient care, including care in psychiatric hospitals and psychiatric units in general hospitals.[68] This ended an era of paying for hospital care on the basis of reimbursement for actual or expected costs. Within one year the provisions of the act proved too rigid and were opposed by the hospital industry for its failure to recognize important differences between hospitals and changes over time in the mix of inpatients in terms of their conditions and the severity of them (the so-called case mix). In 1983, therefore, Congress enacted the Medicare Prospective Payment System (PPS), which implemented a system of paying for each hospital stay at a rate determined prospectively (that is, in advance). Each episode of hospital care was thus paid at an average rate, with the amount adjusted for differences in case mix according to a system of categories called "diagnosis-related groups" or DRGs.[69]

As the result of effective lobbying by the APA and the American Hospital Association, psychiatric specialty inpatient care was excluded from the PPS. Congress mandated that DHHS study the problem of the excluded facilities to determine if the PPS could be applied to these inpatient settings, particularly if the DRGs could be used to adjust for case mix differences among them. Congress called for DHHS to report back to them by the end of 1985. The department assigned responsibility for reporting to Congress to the Health Care Financing Administration (HCFA) and assigned responsibility for the design and conduct of the studies to the Alcohol, Drug Abuse, and Mental Health Administration. NIMH took the lead for the studies within ADAMHA.[70]

ADAMHA convened a work group of interested governmental experts from various agencies affected by the PPS and the excluded facilities.[71] The work group oversaw research contracts designed to address the policy questions. It also expanded to include stakeholders from outside the government. These stakeholders and their organizations in turn developed a series of studies related to the issue—in some cases replicating the government studies. In this fashion the work group provided an opportunity to share data and results from the various studies and to discuss the policy issues. The work group gave the participants a chance to preview the research. Organizations gained a "seat at the table" when they conducted a study. They had an opportunity to influence Congress through their studies, both individually and then collectively through the report to Congress developed by HCFA.[72]

The many studies agreed that there were too many problems in using the DRGs as a case mix measure for adjusting prospective payments to include specialty psychiatric inpatient facilities in the PPS.[73] The various organizations had slightly different interpretations of the findings of their own studies and the government study. HCFA agreed with them all in its central recommendation that the exemption be continued for all psychiatric inpatient admissions except for those in general medical and surgical beds. Participating in the PPS would have produced too many "winners and losers" among the hospitals. Simulations of the impact of the PPS estimated that too many hospitals would suffer large financial losses from being included in the PPS, and too many other hospitals would come away with great profits from the prospective payments. This was considered poor health care financing policy by HCFA, by all of the participants in the work group on PPS, and ultimately by Congress. For the balance of the decade (and in fact until 2005) specialty psychiatric inpatient care would be financed under Medicare according to Tax Equity and Fiscal Responsibility Act rules.[74] At the time this policy of "exceptionalism," special rules for mental health services, was viewed as preferable to full participation in the mainstream PPS of Medicare. Not every policy for improving mental health services called for parity or full participation in mainstream health and social welfare programs with identical policies and rules for inclusion.

Psychiatric inpatient financing policy in Medicare favored a separate, exceptionalist approach; outpatient mental health financing policy favored parity.

Within a decade of the release of the National Plan in 1980 the single Medicare recommendation—to eliminate the $250 dollar limit on outpatient care—was to be implemented and, in fact, considerably exceeded. The first of such changes built upon an unanticipated opportunity that served as an important precedent for Medicare benefit expansions. The opportunity came when the secretary of HHS convened a departmental Task Force on Alzheimer's Disease in 1983.[75] Members of the task force included the assistant secretary of health, Ed Brandt, as chair, and the directors of the National Institute on Aging and the other NIH institutes that were involved in Alzheimer's disease research, including the NIMH. The task force focused principally on biomedical research and only in a limited way on services. Nearing the end of the period of formulating recommendations, the director of NIMH, Herbert Pardes, and the staff director of the task force, Gene Cohen, urged the task force to consider a recommendation to improve mental health coverage in Medicare, which created a barrier to appropriate treatment for Alzheimer's disease patients. The problems included the $250 annual limit and the 50 percent co-payment rate, which were viewed as disincentives for individuals with Alzheimer's disease to receive appropriate treatment for the many troubling behavioral complications of the condition. If a physician used the International Classification of Diseases (ICD) diagnostic codes for Alzheimer's disease that appeared in the mental disorders section of the ICD, rather than the codes in the neurological disease section, then the limits on outpatient treatment for "nervous and mental disease" were applied by Medicare. Individuals with Alzheimer's disease often were seen by psychiatrists for the mental disorder complications of the dementia, such as depression, delusions, and agitation. Psychiatrists, accustomed to using the mental disorder codes from the ICD, recorded these on patients' bills, and Medicare invoked the limitations. Pardes, who had been director of NIMH during the development of the National Plan, saw this opportunity to improve care for individuals with Alzheimer's disease as a vehicle for achieving what the plan had recommended for expanding the mental health benefit in Medicare more broadly.

Brandt and other members of the DHHS leadership felt that a major statutory change affecting all mental disorders was unwise and unlikely to be accomplished. Furthermore, it seemed to them to exceed the mandate of the Task Force on Alzheimer's Disease. Other members of the task force pressed for at least a change for coverage for Alzheimer's disease—to address the specific problems and to create an incremental precedent for improving mental health coverage more broadly. They considered that perhaps a change just for Alzheimer's Disease could be accomplished using HCFA guidelines without more elaborate regulatory or statutory change. HCFA and DHHS were reluctant to make policy changes for a single, specific condition. They had just

experienced legislation creating a special Medicare program for end-stage re-
nal disease and viewed such disorder-specific legislation as problematic and
something they did not wish to repeat. The costs were too high and services
were difficult to regulate.

A series of compromises were worked out among the members of the task
force, the chair, and the task force staff. The first compromise was to focus
only on Alzheimer's disease. The second was to focus only on office visits
rather than on psychotherapy by covering ordinary office visits for treatment
of dementia like any other office visit with respect to co-payments and annual dollar limits in care. Psychotherapy for patients with Alzheimer's disease
generally was uncommon and hence not a major policy concern. Office visits
did not seem to be prone to "moral hazard" and concerns about over-use. The
compromise was finalized at a meeting of the assistant secretary of health, the
assistant secretary for planning and evaluation, and the director of HCFA. At
a moment of some hesitation in the deliberations, it was pointed out that psychiatrists could simply be instructed to use the ICD diagnostic codes used by
neurologists for Alzheimer's disease, and the bill for those services would in-
voke neither the annual limit nor the 50 percent co-payment. This realization
clarified the arbitrary nature of then-current policies and cleared the way for
the policy change. Medicare rules were changed with special instructions to
their carriers that the $250 annual limit and the 50 percent co-payment should
not apply to any outpatient services for medical management of individuals
with a diagnosis of Alzheimer's disease, regardless of which codes were used.
Psychotherapy services would continue to fall under the $250 limit and the 50
percent co-payment rules.

Pardes's prediction that this small change could serve as an important
precedent turned out to be correct—more quickly than expected. Almost immediately there was a series of legislative changes expanding the Medicare mental
health benefit, based in part on the small reform precedent for Alzheimer's disease. The reform was also made possible by the legislative device of this period,
the Omnibus Budget Reconciliation Act, in which hundreds of small legislative
provisions could be combined (and some buried) in a single budget bill each
year. Medicare mental health reform was carried along by the tide of omnibus
legislative bills passed in the mid-1980s.

The first legislative change to the mental health benefit in Medicare in
twenty-two years came in the Omnibus Budget Reconciliation Act of 1987 (PL
100-203).[76] The provisions of the bill increased the maximum annual Medicare
reimbursement from $250 to $1,100. The 50 percent co-payment remained in

place, meaning that Medicare would pay up to $1,100 for $2,200 of outpatient mental health services per year. The law, however, also exempted from the annual limit "medication management visits" to a physician. It set the co-payment rate at 20 percent for these brief office visits for the sole purpose of prescribing or monitoring the effects of psychotropic drugs. This provision built immediately on the distinction made following the deliberations of the Alzheimer's disease task force. It also coincided with growing emphasis on medication treatment in mental health care. The precedent of distinguishing psychotherapy, for which there was concern and evidence about "moral hazard," from other types of outpatient mental health services held sway. Congressional staff were concerned about the breadth and vagueness of the concept of "medical management" that had been at the heart of the Alzheimer's disease task force change in Medicare, and they proposed a more limited exemption from the annual limits and from the 50 percent co-payment for "medication management." This alteration in the original proposal to cover all "medical management" at par was considered non-negotiable. Rather than scuttle the whole reform in Omnibus Budget Reconciliation Act of 1987, mental health advocates felt that this change would again serve as a valuable precedent and was far better than having no reform at all in the mental health benefit in Medicare.[77]

The 1987 legislation also extended coverage to "hospital based and hospital affiliated" partial hospitalization services.[78] These were intensive services for patients who did not need the restrictions of an inpatient hospital but needed more services than could be provided in traditional outpatient visits. These programs were connected to hospitals, and while they had been shown to be cost-effective substitutes for hospital stays for carefully selected patients, partial hospital programs could also expand services to individuals who did not need the intensive level of care provided in a partial hospital. Congress acted almost immediately to cover only programs operated by hospitals as of January 1989, excluding many CMHCs from coverage of their partial hospitalization programs. This restriction appeared first as technical amendments to PL 100-203 and then attached to the Medicare Catastrophic Coverage Act of 1988 (PL 100-360). The budget legislation of 1987 also provided payments to clinical psychologists, even when there was no physician supervision, if they were working in community mental health centers or rural health clinics.

The final change in Medicare for the 1980s was dramatic. The Omnibus Budget Reconciliation Act of 1989 (101-239) removed the annual limit entirely for all services, including psychotherapy. It also extended coverage to psychologists and social workers that were Medicare-authorized providers. The legislation also reversed the technical restrictions on partial hospital services, permitting reimbursement in all CHMCs that were licensed to provided partial hospitalization and that provided it as one of the "essential services," as defined by the Public Health Service requirements for centers. The act, however, did not remove the 50 percent co-payment for outpatient treatment for "nervous and mental disorders" other than for "medication management." This restriction has remained unchanged as of this writing. Efforts to achieve parity coverage for Medicare have paralleled other such legislative advocacy for parity in private health insurance.

Through a series of strategic incremental steps, guided by the single recommendation of the National Plan, Medicare's mental health benefit dramatically improved, far exceeding the expectations of the plan.

Conventional wisdom argues that federal mental health policy entered a dark age with the rise of the Reagan revolution and the twelve years of Republican domination of the executive branch and growth in conservative power in legislative and judicial branches as well. Certainly many of the changes in social policy had damaging effects on individuals with severe and persistent mental disorders. The almost immediate passage of Omnibus Budget Reconciliation Act of 1981 reinforced the new approach to federalism in which the role of the federal government waned in favor of states and localities. The act repealed virtually all of the Mental Health Systems Act, dashing the enthusiasm for major reform that characterized the Carter years and the PCMH. In addition it repealed the CMHC Act. There were no initiatives for growth in federal support of mental health services. On the contrary, the block grants that replaced the CMHC Act grants diminished federal categorical support for mental health services and fell far short of the expectations of the Mental Health Systems Act and the recommendations of the PCMH.

The Community Support Program and the National Plan were the sole survivors of the reform that placed individuals with severe and persistent mental disorders at the top of the priority list with the recognition that mental health policy flowed in the mainstream of general health and social welfare policy.[79] It involved housing, employment, and transportation policy as well as income support, disability, and health care financing policy. Advocates, only temporarily daunted by the turn in political favors, used the plan as a blueprint for incremental reforms through the 1980s, achieving a measure of "quiet success." The sequential reforms brought significant changes to the

Social Security disability programs, SSI and SSDI, as well as to Medicaid and Medicare. The reforms in SSI and SSDI increased the rolls of people with mental disability and made it easier for individuals with mental impairments to gain access to their entitlements. These income benefits were the key to independent living outside of institutions and in the community for millions of disabled individuals, and they also provided eligibility to health insurance, through Medicaid and Medicare.

In contrast to the conventional wisdom, the 1980s saw many progressive advances in federal mental health policy—at least as measured against the policy aspirations of the National Plan. A substantial majority of the recommendations of the plan had been implemented by 1991. These policy reforms in the federal health care financing programs changed the face of mental health services for decades to come. Medicaid and Medicare were to eclipse state categorical dollars as a source of mental health services funding in the 1990s. While the new federalism made states even more important in mental health services policy, the federal government was to pick up more of the bill.

For all of the successes of mental health policy in the 1980s, policies and programs remained fragmented.[80] Federal agencies in charge of the entitlement programs were separated by bureaucratic walls within DHHS and among the other federal departments with some influence on the lives of individuals experiencing a mental disorder, including HUD and the Departments of Labor and Education. There was limited communication between the SSA and the HCFA and with the NIMH. A range of new social problems involving people with mental illness, such as homelessness and HIV/AIDS, created new pressures for reform of the fragmented mental health system. Medicaid and Medicare may have improved mental health benefits, but these benefits had more limitations than those for general health services did. Nor was there parity for mental health coverage in the employer-sponsored health insurance market that covered most Americans (although parity for individuals with severe and persistent mental disorders was less pressing, if only because virtually none were employed and hence nearly all lacked insurance coverage). And if most people were underinsured for mental health care, the growing ranks of uninsured individuals placed increasing demands on the public mental health system as well as on other institutions, such as public hospitals and their emergency rooms and the criminal justice system. The system was fragmented: no one agency accepted responsibility. People with mental disorders were often the victims of discrimination in housing opportunities, in employment, and in health insurance. Advocates called for integration, parity, and a transformation of mental health policy.

Chapter 6

Integration, Parity, and Transformation

While federal mental health policy was "inching forward" in the 1980s, the fragmentation of the mental health system intensified. Policy advances followed the recommendations of the National Plan for the Chronically Mentally Ill to make sequential changes in the Social Security Administration disability programs, notably Medicare and in Medicaid. Access to mainstream benefits improved, but that meant that the mental health system of the 1990s had even more diverse sources of revenue and many more regulations to follow than in the 1980s.

As individuals with severe and persistent mental disorders spent more and more time in their communities, they found themselves in an ever-widening range of social institutions. They were involved with public housing, employment services and vocational rehabilitation programs, schools, and increasingly in the criminal justice system. All of these institutions and agencies were responsible, but there was no centralized accountability. The traditional state mental health system no longer provided all of the resources needed by the individuals for whom they had responsibility. Medicaid expansions in the 1980s were controlled in most instances not by the state mental health authorities but rather by a separate Medicaid agency. Local governments shared responsibility through their involvement with mental health services and with the many other institutions where people with mental health problems sought care and treatment or caused problems because their needs were different and their behaviors were challenging.[1]

The NIMH Community Support Program had focused attention on these problems in the 1970s, but lost momentum during the 1980s. The CSP had fought a successful rear-guard action during the 1980s, and remained a model as well as a focal point for slow reform. Nevertheless, it was unable to meet the growing need for a policy approach that was designed to overcome service fragmentation. Although the National Plan had identified fragmentation as a key problem with the system, it did not offer a viable solution to this thorny issue.[2]

Services integration along with organizational coordination and collaboration had been the main strategies to overcome the problem of fragmentation since the 1960s. The CMHCs relied on these mechanisms to bring a range of mental health services under one service umbrella. The expansion of the target population of CMHCs and the range of required services challenged continuity of care and integration of services even further.[3] The CSP offered an innovative model for dealing with fragmentation for individuals with the most disabling conditions, but when homelessness emerged as a major social problem in the 1980s the need to coordinate mental health and social welfare services became even more acute.[4] Several demonstration programs from the late 1980s and throughout the 1990s tested a variety of models of service integration. The results of the evaluations of these demonstration projects ended up shifting attention from an exclusive reliance on organizational and financing strategies to a focus on the content and quality of care.[5] (The focus on effective treatments and evidence-based practices emerges as a major theme in the 1990s in a series of projects and demonstration programs discussed below. It also proved critical in improvements in insurance coverage for mental health care.)

The federal agencies responsible for providing a focus on mental health services themselves underwent organizational reform that only exacerbated policy fragmentation. Once housed together within NIMH, the federal research, services, and policy functions were divided in 1992. The NIMH research activities returned to the National Institutes of Health (from its separate home in the Alcohol, Drug Abuse, and Mental Health Administration in DHHS), and the Substance Abuse and Mental Health Services Administration (SAMHSA) was created in DHHS for the service and policy functions.

Some of the demonstration programs were partnerships between federal and state governments, and others were public–private partnerships. Private foundations began to involve themselves in mental health policy and services, thus challenging the mental health services field with new ideas. But while resources from public sources diversified and expanded during the 1980s and 1990s and Medicare and Medicaid moved toward parity, private insurance coverage remained unequal and discriminatory.[6] Advocates pushed not only for full parity in Medicare but also for parity in state insurance laws, for priority for federal employees, and for a federal parity law affecting self-insured plans, which were otherwise exempt from state regulations. During the 1990s the sequential changes in the public financing programs that had occurred in the 1980s began to affect the private sector as well. This expansion was hastened by the rise of managed care and the potential to control the costs associated with benefit expansions. The health care reforms of the 1990s—successful and unsuccessful—advanced the role of managed care and considered mental health and substance abuse services within the mandates of those reforms. Model mental health benefits were proposed and challenged, but the debate over mental health services was no longer postponed or isolated from the broad, mainstream reform of health care policy.[7]

At the end of the 1990s a White House conference on mental health was followed by the release of the first-ever report on mental health by the surgeon general.[8] Both had been pushed by Tipper Gore, the wife of the vice president, who had also co-chaired the Workgroup on Mental Health for the health care reform process.[9] When Al Gore lost the contested election of 2000 and George W. Bush became president, many mental health advocates felt a particular loss, since the assumption was that a Gore administration would have been very supportive of mental health. The fear was that the momentum associated with the excitement of the end-of-the-century mental health landmark decisions would be lost. The situation was somewhat similar to the defeat of Carter, who, with his wife, had championed mental health. Yet the loss of the presidency to Ronald Reagan, who cared little about mental health policy, had been followed by surprising incremental successes during the Reagan–Bush years. Furthermore, the new President Bush promised a mental health commission and called for a transformation of many government approaches to firmly entrenched social problems.

Would the sequential advances of the 1980s and the drive for integration and parity give way to a fundamental redirection of mental health services in the new century? Would there be a long-awaited transformation of federal mental health policy?

When Ronald Reagan took office, federal mental health policy debates went underground.[10] While advocates worked with Congress to reshape the mainstream federal entitlement programs according to the recommendations of the National Plan, the center of the action moved to the states—to state mental health authorities in particular. The National Plan was anathema to the new administration, which advocated, at least in theory, a sharp diminution in federal social, welfare, and medical responsibilities. At the NIMH the CSP and its analogue for children—the Child and Adolescent Service System Program—continued to provide some federal leadership by urging state mental health authorities to create community support systems. The problem of fragmented services, however, remained as pressing as ever, and services integration remained the principal focus of the NIMH efforts at innovation. [11]

"Systems integration" was a strategy of bringing together a service system that provided all of the diverse services needed for individuals who experienced a severe and persistent mental disorder.[12] The goal was to build a "community support system" at the state and local level. That meant building collaborative linkages among the respective agencies responsible for those services, such as housing, welfare, schools, and the criminal and juvenile justice agencies. The overall strategy seemed to make sense on its face, although earlier manifestations of systems integration in programs, such as Model Cities in the War on Poverty, had been criticized as failures. Studies of these programs concluded that it was not in the nature of organizations to cooperate and to be integrated. Furthermore, it was difficult to identify the precise attributes of the community support system that the NIMH's program promoted, and the effectiveness of many of the mental health services of the era (other than the psychoactive medications and electroconvulsive treatment) had yet to be documented. In spite of efforts by the new administration to eliminate the CSP, the Congress retained the program in the NIMH appropriation bill year after year, and the agency continued its efforts to fund grants for systems integration activities within the state mental health authorities. With the demise of the CMHC program in 1981 and its replacement with the Alcohol, Drug Abuse, and Mental Health Services Block Grant, services and service system development at the local level became the responsibility of the states and not the federal government.

Early in the Reagan years, the CSP turned its attention to a new social problem that disproportionately affected individuals with mental illness—homelessness in the nation's urban areas.[13] Newspapers and other media focused attention on this new social problem. The sudden rise in homelessness was a complex phenomenon not easily explained. Some attributed the rise in the homeless population to the gentrification of cities and decline in single-room occupancy residences and other low-rent housing. Some placed responsibility upon the deinstitutionalization of people with severe mental disorders. Experts, the media, and mental health advocates argued that failure to provide community mental health services that were designed to support individuals in the new era of deinstitutionalization never materialized, and the disability policies of the new administration only exacerbated the problem.

The Robert Wood Johnson Foundation (RWJF) moved to fill the void created by the failure of the federal government to address the problem of homelessness. The RWJF—by far the largest private health philanthropic foundation—developed a program called Health Care for the Homeless to provide health care and support services for individuals who were homeless in cities across the country. Guided by foundation vice president Linda Aiken, the program quickly identified large numbers of individuals with severe mental disorders among the homeless population. The mental health literature was filled with reports of this growing problem. Aiken, together with RWJF advisor and health and social policy expert David Mechanic, pressed for more attention to the special problem of homelessness and mental illness. Until that time, RWJF had excluded mental health issues from its philanthropic programs. Nevertheless, the RWJF found it impossible to ignore the issue of fragmented mental health services if it was to continue to address the problem of homelessness.[14]

The specific problem identified by Aiken and Mechanic was the lack of a locus of responsibility and authority for individuals with mental health problems at the local level.[15] Cities or counties rarely had an effective local mental health authority that could respond to a request from homelessness service agencies to provide assistance and services for an individual with a severe mental illness. There was nowhere for either the individual or the agency to turn. Frustration was accompanied by neglect. There was no single point of clinical, fiscal or administrative accountability for individuals who were homeless and experienced a severe mental illness. Aiken and Mechanic convinced the RWJF to take on the problem of mental health services in large urban areas. The foundation developed three programs in mental illness. Between 1984 and 1986 its staff explored various ideas. They communicated with experts in the field, including NIMH staff. At the outset the NIMH manifested some hesitancy for a variety of putative reasons. There was some competitiveness between the foundation and a federal agency, if only because the entry of a private organization implied that government efforts were not successful. Furthermore, the approaches suggested by the foundation challenged some of the basic assumptions of CSP. The focus of the RWJF programs was on local rather than state government, and some of the attention was on direct service development and not just service system integration.[16]

Two of the three new programs did focus almost entirely on fragmentation and promoted systems integration concepts; the third program—the Mental

Health Services Development Program—funded local service innovations. Leonard Stein, a professor of psychiatry at the University of Wisconsin, directed the third program. Stein was an innovator in mental health services and had developed and established the effectiveness of assertive community treatment (ACT). ACT was an early "evidence-based practice." It involved a multidisciplinary team with a small caseload that provided intensive mental health services to individuals wherever they were in the community without requiring that they attend office appointments. It was effective in reducing hospitalizations, and its clients returned to work more often than those who were in comparative community treatment settings. The Mental Health Services Development Program made grant awards to local communities to develop specialized mental health services such as ACT as well as rehabilitation services. At the time the program was viewed as more prosaic than the other two systems integration programs, but as time went on the content of care and evidence-based practices were of increasing interest and importance.

The two other programs—the Mental Health Services Program for Youth and the Program on Chronic Mental Illness—both focused on systems integration. They were intended to demonstrate the merits of centralizing authority and responsibility for services for young people with severe emotional disturbance and for adults with severe and persistent mental disorders. The Mental Health Services Program for Youth, directed by Mary Jane England, a child psychiatrist and public services administrator, and Robert F. Cole, a child mental health expert, involved a wide array of human services providers in a network of integrated services designed to meet the needs of children with severe emotional disorders in urban areas. These systems of care placed parents and their children at the center of a system that included the schools and juvenile justice and child welfare agencies, as well as more traditional child-serving health and mental health services. The larger Program on Chronic Mental Illness, directed by psychiatrist Miles Shore and social worker Martin Cohen, had a similar intent but focused explicitly on developing a local mental health authority as the mechanism for organizing and financing mental health services for adults with severe mental illness in large urban areas.[17]

The Program on Chronic Mental Illness was launched late in 1986, when the RWJF provided $29 million in grants and loans to nine of the largest cities in the nation—Austin, Baltimore, Charlotte, Cincinnati, Columbus, Denver, Honolulu, Philadelphia, and Toledo. Augmenting these awards, the Department of Housing and Urban Development provided each city with 125 Section 8 certificates, permitting the local mental health authorities to subsidize rents for persons with severe mental illnesses. Shore and Cohen established a national program office at Harvard Medical School to dispense technical assistance to local mental health authorities dealing with mental health services and low-cost housing.[18]

The Program on Chronic Mental Illness emphasized the creation of local mental health authorities as the vehicle for overcoming the problems of service and policy fragmentation.[19] Many problems derived from a disjuncture between local needs and the state and federal policies and programs that provided re-sources to meet those needs. Hence the program recommended the creation of a local structure that would take responsibility for individuals with chronic mental illness living in community settings. The local mental health authority was ex-pected to centralize administrative, clinical, and fiscal responsibility in a single entity. The logic of the demonstration then postulated that an effective authority would be able to organize and finance mental health services and coordinate the other needs of individuals with chronic mental illness, particularly their hous-ing needs. That was the most important innovation and the critical new resource offered by the Program on Chronic Mental Illness, namely, the opportunity to use Section 8 certificates and thus demonstrate that individuals with even the most disabling mental disorders could use such rental subsidies to live in ordi-nary community housing, if given appropriate services and supports.

The Program on Chronic Mental Illness was a systems change intervention focused on organizing and financing care rather than on providing resources for direct services. The expectation was that better-run local mental health authori-ties would allocate existing resources (or newly gained Medicaid resources for eligible clients) for direct services. At the end of the start-up phase of the dem-onstration, however, a group of clinician members of the National Advisory Committee appointed by the Robert Wood Johnson Foundation made a series of site visits and returned with doubts about the potential for the success of the program. They argued forcefully that most of the sites had little or no clinical leadership or expertise and that clinical authority was not sufficiently devel-oped to make the projects effective. At the time their criticism was only partly heard. There were efforts to develop clinical service plans in each city under the direction of the local mental health authority, but many leaders in the Pro-gram on Chronic Mental Illness felt that senior clinicians overvalued clinical work and did not really "understand" the service integration concepts at the heart of the demonstration.[20] The evaluation of the Program on Chronic Illness would end up addressing this issue, and it became central to the national poli-cy debate during succeeding years.

Together the RWJF and the NIMH developed a plan for an elaborate evaluation of the Program on Chronic Mental Illness.[21] The proposed study was the largest and most complex evaluation in the foundation's history. Although the NIMH's CSP had not been involved in the development of and planning for the Program on Chronic Mental Illness, the new services research component of the NIMH, under the direction of Carl A. Taube, offered to play an important role in the evaluation. The NIMH agreed to fund half of the cost of the multiyear study and to oversee the review of the nine proposals submitted in response to a competitive solicitation. Each organization allocated $2 million to the effort.

Taube considered the evaluation of the Program on Chronic Mental Illness as a unique opportunity to test the evolving science of mental health services research in a study that would combine an investigation of service system implementation activities and their relationship to client-level outcomes. Originally the RWJF wanted only to evaluate the implementation of the systems-level intervention and focus on the local mental health authorities. The NIMH, however, insisted on assessing client outcomes in terms of symptomatology, functioning, and quality of life. The evaluation was multifaceted, and consequently the study team was composed of individuals with expertise in clinical services, family burden, interorganizational networks, financing, and housing. The proposed comprehensive design of the evaluation substantially exceeded the budget of $4 million, and the investigators submitted additional grant proposals to the NIMH that were funded separately. This funding enabled the entire project to go forward.

What did the evaluation ultimately reveal? The results were complex and confusing to many people, including the foundation staff, many of whom believed that the evaluation had concluded that the Program on Chronic Mental Illness was a failure.[22] They focused on the main outcome findings—that the outcomes of the cohorts of clients who were observed late in the demonstration improved no more than the outcomes of the clients who were observed early in the demonstration. On average the clients improved in both time periods, but the improvements during the period of maximum involvement of the local mental health authorities were no greater than those observed nearer to the beginning of their implementation. This part of the evaluation indicated that either the most important effects of the demonstration occurred so early in the implementation process that the evaluators missed them or that the local mental health authorities had little impact on the groups of clients selected for more detailed study. Most observers concluded that the local mental health authorities had little impact on clients of their respective systems in spite of more service system integration over the course of the demonstration.

These negative findings dominated all other findings for many observers of the Program on Chronic Mental Illness, even though the evaluation was otherwise quite positive. The various component studies within the evaluation indicated that the local mental health authorities were either created from scratch or—where they existed prior to the demonstration—increased their centralized responsibility. The demonstration was associated with increased interorganizational integration and the development in each city of new agencies to expand housing opportunities for clients and to use the HUD Section 8 certificates.[23] Financing changes encouraged the use of Medicaid, and new state government incentives to treat individuals with severe and persistent mental illness also led to increases in local funding for treating mental illness.[24] The Program on Chronic Mental Illness demonstrated the feasibility and utility of the local mental health authorities as a means of improving the system of care.[25] Nevertheless, doubts lingered about the impact on individuals with severe mental illness. One component of the evaluation found that later in the demonstration clients were more likely to have case managers (that is, individuals who provided emotional support and assisted them with making sure that they received appropriate care) and to have continuity of care.[26] Another component study showed that families of the clients who had case managers experienced less objective and subjective "burden."[27] Lastly, individuals who lived in their own apartments using Section 8 rent subsidies and who had case managers did show clinical improvements and gains in quality of life.[28] Clearly there were some positive individual outcomes and benefits for clients who used services in Program on Chronic Mental Illness cities.

The evaluators themselves concluded that the local mental health authorities may have been necessary to improve the system of care for individuals with a chronic mental illness, but that the change in the system was not sufficient to produce good outcomes.[29] They began to focus on the content and quality of the services received by the clients directly, speculating that many of the services delivered in the Program on Chronic Mental Illness cities were not the "evidence-based" services, such as assertive community treatment, whose effectiveness had been established through research.[30]

However one views the outcomes of the Program on Chronic Mental Illness, the demonstration reflected a receptivity toward changes in thinking about strategies to improve care and treatment of individuals with severe mental disorders. During the early years of the CSP, the emphasis had been on changes in the system of care. In the 1990s, by contrast, the focus began to shift to the quality of services and evidence-based practices. Other demonstration projects at the same time came to similar conclusions about the merits of systems change.[31] Although the RWJF demonstration program for youth did not measure individual outcomes at all, several other demonstration programs for children raised questions about what came to be called the "systems change hypothesis."[32] Investigators and sponsors of demonstration programs began to look more deeply at the direct services being provided to adults with severe and persistent mental disorders and children with serious emotional disturbances.[33]

The findings of the evaluation of the Program on Chronic Mental Illness as well as other studies that raised questions about the "systems integration hypothesis" shaped the next generation of mental health service demonstrations coming from the federal government. Although lagging behind the private foundation sector in its response to the problems of homelessness and mental illness, by the late 1980s the NIMH, the National Institute on Alcohol Abuse and Alcoholism (NIAAA), and the National Institute on Drug Abuse (NIDA) (the three component ADAMHA institutes) all developed programs under the Stewart B. McKinney Homeless Assistance Act.[34] This piece of legislation authorized and appropriated resources to develop service demonstration programs for homeless individuals and to evaluate them. Although service fragmentation was identified as a problem to be addressed in programs for homeless individuals with mental and addictive disorders, the McKinney Act demonstrations focused principally on direct service interventions rather than on systems change. However, these demonstration programs in diverse sites across the nation did not specify services to be delivered, and it was difficult to make valid comparisons among the various project sites. The federal government did not want to interfere with local innovation and in keeping with the principles of the new federalism, did not want to impose many requirements on local government and private-sector efforts. Much was learned from individual site studies, but little could be gleaned from the cross-site evaluation efforts.

As the Program on Chronic Mental Illness and several of the McKinney Act demonstration projects were ending in 1992, a Bush administration federal task force on homelessness and mental illness delivered its report. *Outcasts on Main Street* called for a demonstration program to test the systems integration hypothesis for reducing homelessness among individuals with a severe mental illness.[35] The program proposed to assess whether a comparatively small amount of money (about $100,000 each year) to implement a series of service integration activities, such as co-locating services and pooling funding, would promote better cooperation among mental health and other human service providers. In the experimental sites the $100,000 grants were to be included in the larger grants for services.The evaluation would then determine whether these enhancements to the system of care would in turn improve the housing status and quality of life of homeless mentally ill individuals. The program was called ACCESS (Access to Community Care and Effective Services and Supports), and it was influenced by the experiences of the RWJF's Program on Chronic Mental Illness and of the McKinney Act demonstrations.[36]

Implemented in 1993, the ACCESS program was different in several respects from its predecessors. Unlike the McKinney Act projects, there was a renewed focus on integration of services. Like the RWJF Program on Chronic Mental Illness, the ACCESS program proposed to test the systems integration hypothesis, while directly providing evidence-based services at each project site. Nine states were selected to participate in ACCESS; each state proposed two sites. Unlike the RWJF Program on Chronic Mental Illness, each of the eighteen program sites was given a direct service grant of between $600,000 and $800,000 to implement and maintain an assertive community treatment (ACT) team, an evidence-based service. One site in each state was selected at random to additionally receive a small grant to promote services integration activities. The theory of the demonstration was to determine if the addition of resources to integrate services would lead to changes in the organization and coordination of care in the nine grantee cities and whether these changes would lead to improvements in the outcomes of individual clients of the ACT teams. Unlike the McKinney Act demonstrations, all of the sites participated in an elaborate evaluation design that had been predetermined and was a precondition of receiving the ACCESS grants.

As in the RWJF Program on Chronic Mental Illness, the evaluation of the ACCESS program demonstrated that resources directed at service integration activities produced some of their intended effects at the program sites that received the added grant resources.[37] The effects on individual clients were less clear.[38] There was some indication that previously homeless individuals in the better-integrated sites were more likely to be independently housed twelve months after starting ACT services. Overall the evaluation of the ACCESS program concluded that service systems integration could not be depended upon to produce broad improvements in client outcomes, but the evaluators suggested that sites appeared to appreciate some of the administrative benefits of better-integrated systems.[39] The evaluation reinforced the importance of delivering direct, evidence-based services, such as ACT, to improve the outcomes of homeless mentally ill individuals in large urban areas. The study emphasized the need for effective clinical services and supports for adults—even in better-integrated service systems. During this same period, however, children's mental health services continued to emphasize systems of care, although there was some recognition of the importance of providing effective services as well.[40] The field was moving slowly away from a reliance on systems integration as the main force for change, and the service system remained fragmented in most communities.

Federal mental health policy subtly followed, or at least reflected, the new trend to focus on the content and quality of care. One of the first opportunities to refocus attention came in 1992, almost immediately on the heels of the Program on Chronic Mental Illness, in the form of a contract from the federal agency then called the Agency for Health Care Policy and Research (AHCPR), later called the Agency for Healthcare Research and Quality (AHRQ). The contract was for a Patient Outcome Research Team on Schizophrenia.[41] The team was a mechanism employed by AHCPR to study patient outcomes for various conditions—to review the effectiveness of treatments, to study patterns of care, and to develop and disseminate treatment recommendations. Donald Steinwachs at the Johns Hopkins University School of Public Health and Anthony Lehman at the University of Maryland School of Medicine, both of whom were members of the RWJF Program on Chronic Mental Illness evaluation team, directed the Schizophrenia outcome research team from 1992 to 1998.

The team established more broadly what Program on Chronic Mental Illness investigators had observed less systematically in the nine demonstration cities that mental health systems were not providing recommended care for patients with schizophrenia. The Patient Outcome Research Team found that the evidence on effectiveness was considerable, but that such evidence was not affecting actual practice.[42]

The findings of a gap between research and practice influenced various aspects of federal mental health policy in the late 1990s and into the next century. The focus on implementing evidence-based practices grew with the publication of several reports including *Mental Health—A Report of the Surgeon General*

(1999) and the Final Report of the President's New Freedom Commission on Mental Health, *Achieving the Promise: Transforming Mental Health Care in America* (2003).[43] The findings also led to another public–private collaboration. The partnership between the RWJF and SAMHSA on the Evidence-Based Practices Project, based at the New Hampshire–Dartmouth Psychiatric Research Center, began in 2000 under the direction of Robert E. Drake at Dartmouth Medical School.[44] This project developed a series of implementation resource kits that were then used to assist eight states in implementing a set of evidence-based practices for adults with severe mental disorders. The set of six practices was selected by a team of investigators and Laurie Flynn of the National Alliance for the Mentally Ill (NAMI). The investigators included Drake and members of the Schizophrenia Patient Outcome Research Team, carrying forward the observations that had their roots in the limitations of the services integration hypothesis.

As the Reagan–Bush years came to a close in 1992, two phases of federal mental health policy shifted and a new trend began. The decade of "quiet success" and piecemeal, sequential changes in policies governing mental health in mainstream programs such as Medicare, Medicaid, SSI, and SSDI slowly gave way to a more open acceptance of mental health care as an element of federal health policy in the Clinton administration. In addition, the focus on systems change was gradually augmented by a concern for the effectiveness of direct care services for treatment and rehabilitation. The watershed year for federal mental health policy came in 1992. In that year the RWJF Program on Chronic Mental Illness officially ended, *Outcasts on Main Street* was released, the ACCESS program was initiated, and the schizophrenia outcome research team began its activities. The Clinton-Gore election also brought changes in federal mental health policy.

At about this time a new strategy for handling health care costs emerged. Managed care offered a case-by-case review of appropriateness of care coupled with hard-negotiated prices and prospectively set rates as a way of damping the explosion in health care costs.[45] Managed care was to figure prominently in discussions of mental health policy for the next decade or more. When Clinton won the presidency in 1992 health care policy had become a major national issue, and the Clinton-Gore transition team went to work on health care reform. Mental health care became an element in that policy debate, then and in the decade-long wake of its disappointing outcome.

———————

Clinton's election was greeted with considerable enthusiasm by mental health advocates, not so much for any specific mental health policy promises that the new president had made but because there was hope that he would include mental health care in the forecasted health care reform proposals. This optimism was reinforced by the election of his vice presidential running mate, Al Gore, whose wife, Tipper, was a known advocate for mental health. Tipper Gore had been active in a group of congressional spouses interested in mental health issues at the same time that her husband served in the Senate. The Clinton-Gore health care transition team included a number of individuals with an interest in mental health services. The initial discussions of health care reform, however, never reached the level of detail about the proposed benefit design. Shortly after the inauguration excitement died down, the Health Care Reform Task Force was formed. Tipper Gore was appointed co-chair of a Work Group on Mental Health and Substance Abuse; Bernard Arons, a psychiatrist on the staff at NIMH, was appointed as the other co-chair of the work group. Arons, who worked on health care financing issues at the institute, had just finished a fellowship spent on the Hill.[46]

The work group included a group of federal employees from NIMH, NIDA, and NIAAA, staff from AHCPR and the newly created SAMHSA, as well as a small group of individuals who held federal grants and expert-consultant appointments with various agencies. An occasional Hill staff person also joined the work group, but most of the participants were longtime federal bureaucrats or federal consultants. Almost everyone on the work group brimmed with enthusiasm and hoped that the group's recognition as a regular component of the health care reform process meant that mental health benefits would be included in the standard benefit package that was to stand at the center of the reform.

The deliberations of the Work Group on Mental Health and Substance Abuse began in Little Rock, Arkansas, in early February 1993. Shortly thereafter the weekly meetings moved to the Old Executive Office Building adjacent to the White House and continued through the end of April. By that time the Health Security Act had been drafted, and there was no reason for the Work Group to continue meeting regularly. Mental health and substance abuse services were included in the benefit design, but the advocates did not get everything that they wanted. When health care reform failed along with the bill, there was widespread disappointment, but the inclusion of mental health benefits was a sort of rhetorical victory and another incremental success for federal mental health policy.

Many revealing things happened in the few short months of the health care reform process from the early February meetings in Little Rock to the special White House reception in May, offered as a thank-you to work group members. The activities of the work group and the issues it considered in 1993 foreshadowed federal mental health policy as it would evolve over the next decade. As much as the events of health care reform looked forward to the next ten years, the deliberations and ultimate design of the mental health benefit had their foundations in earlier mental health services research sponsored by the federal government.

Carl Taube at NIMH (and later at the Johns Hopkins University School of Public Health) had spent most of the decade developing the field of mental health services research and mental health economics. When he died prematurely in 1989 at the age of fifty, Taube left a body of research and a broader capacity to study the effects of financing policies. Under his guidance NIMH had conducted or sponsored extensive research on prospective payment and studies of patterns of outpatient practice, as well as analyses of demand for mental health services under various health insurance arrangements. *Health Affairs*—a young but increasingly influential journal—published a series of papers on mental health financing in 1990 and again in 1992, all of which were used in the health care reform debates.[47] The emerging research on the early efforts in managed behavioral health care, such as the Civilian Health and Medical Program of the Uniformed Services (CHAMPUS) Tidewater demonstration, also figured in the discussion of mechanisms to control costs if insurance coverage for mental health and substance abuse services were to be expanded. The Department of Defense had initiated the use of managed behavioral health care for CHAMPUS in the Tidewater of Virginia, which showed that it was possible to curtail costs dramatically, especially by reducing the use of expensive hospital stays and days.[48]

The two main issues impeding the expansion of mental health and substance abuse coverage in health insurance were lack of confidence in the effectiveness of treatment for mental disorders and concerns about costs.[49] At worst, opponents of increased insurance coverage for mental disorders dismissed the mental health conditions themselves as trivial and lacking in scientific foundation. Even when some opponents of improved coverage would concede that mental disorders were real health conditions, they doubted that treatment would produce reproducible benefits. Furthermore, if the conditions were not "real" and individuals sought treatment as a matter of choice rather than need, then mental health treatment was not an insurable event.

Even if it was an insurable event, other critics believed that there was substantial "moral hazard" associated with use of insurance; that is, the price-lowering effect of insurance would stimulate demand for mental health services to an extent greater than it already did for general medical services. In economic terms the demand for mental health services was more "price elastic" than for other similar services, making it a problem for improving coverage, especially if the insurance coverage did not require higher cost-sharing requirements (for example, co-payments, limits, or deductibles) to dampen demand.

The federally funded RAND Health Insurance Experiment from the 1970s and a range of other nonexperimental studies all sustained the view that there was a moral hazard problem, absent some other control on utilization.[50] The studies found that the demand for mental health services was about twice as price responsive as the demand for all other general medical services in the aggregate. That is, when general medical care went from being paid out of pocket to being covered nearly in full, utilization doubled. Utilization quadrupled for outpatient mental health services under full insurance.[51] To compound the problem, mental health insurance was also subject to "adverse selection." Individuals with persistent mental disorders knew that they needed and planned to use mental health services at the beginning of each year. Following clear economic incentives and their health care needs, individuals already diagnosed with a mental disorder tended to enroll in plans that offered them better insurance coverage for mental health treatment. As a result, plans such as the High Option federal employees' plans that historically offered excellent mental health benefits attracted a concentration of heavy users of mental health services.[52]

Mandating coverage of mental disorders in all insurance plans underwritten in a state or under the control of the federal government has been used as one way of controlling adverse selection. If all plans have the same benefit structure, then no individual will move from one plan to another because of benefit differences or advantages. Nevertheless, mandated coverage, does not help with the moral hazard problem; managed care, however, potentially does deal with the need to control costs through various forms of utilization review. Managed care can make improved mental health benefits possible—at least in terms of providing a brake against the incentive for demand to rise when insurance coverage improves. But although managed care offered an option for expanding insurance coverage for mental health treatment, there was considerable opposition to managed behavioral health care. Clinicians who provided mental health services often opposed managed care as an intrusion on their clinical judgment and a restraint on their professional practices. Some service users also considered it an intrusion in terms of reporting personal health information to a third party and also a limitation on choice of provider. Using managed care to achieve better insurance coverage was perceived by some as a "Faustian bargain."

This was the state of mental health financing when the broader debate began to consider the inclusion of mental health and substance abuse services in the benefit package in health care reform. In 1993 mainstream policymakers were concerned about the insurability of mental health services. Although eventually there was substantial evidence about the cost-saving potential for managed care, in 1993 policymakers (and the actuaries who predicted what their policy ideas would cost) doubted how effective managed care would be in solving the moral hazard problem.[53]

The euphoria of the initial meetings of the Work Group on Mental Health and Substance Abuse was expressed in terms of expansive ideas about benefit design and service system reform without any apparent concern about the dual realities of economic scarcity and political opposition.[54] Discussion waxed eloquent about the need for expanded mental health and substance abuse services in the private sector, preventive services and new systems of care in the public sector. It was assumed that the work group would develop a "parity benefit" equal in every respect to the general medical benefits in terms of cost-sharing provisions and limits. Most members of the Work Group dismissed as "old thinking" comments about the realities of cost containment and past political opponents who still did not believe that mental disorders were real health conditions or that mental health treatment was effective. The work group reflected a more widespread sense that the health care reform process had a mandate to break from past precedents.

The work group deliberated under this enthusiastic direction and produced a rich "parity" benefit design with all of the facets favored by mental health advocates. Policies were also developed for public mental health systems redesign and maintenance of effort from state mental health authorities. When this design work reached the stage of sufficient specificity, it was subjected to "scoring" by the actuaries. Richard Frank, a health economist from Harvard Medical School and an authority on mental health financing, consulted to the work group and collaborated with the other economists and actuaries involved more broadly in the health care reform process.

The process was laid out in a series of stages, called "tollgates" through which each iteration of the proposal needed to pass. The benefit design was discussed on March 19, 1993, at "Tollgate 4" with the senior members of the

Health Care Reform Task Force. While the basic approach was given a green light, the mental health and substance abuse benefit was to be implemented in stages. The first benefit in the legislation would be more limited than parity, similar to what had been proposed previously in the NIMH project on model benefits and reported in the *Health Affairs* papers.[55] Psychotherapy would be limited with higher co-payments, and other service limits would be imposed. A parity benefit would be introduced only in the next stage of health care reform. Essentially the actuaries did not accept that the managed care structures and techniques that would be in place in the proposed "managed competition" arrangements for the reformed health care system would be adequate to control costs due to the increase in demand associated with parity insurance coverage. This decision modified the euphoria of the work group, but there was appreciation that the standard benefit design would include mental health and substance abuse benefits.

Members of the work group also were excited that they would brief the president and vice president on March 20 on their work. Many other high-ranking federal officials were included at the White House presentation, including cabinet secretaries and their deputies from the DHHS and Department of Labor, as well as the Council of Economic Advisers and the President's chief of staff. Although this was probably the highest-level federal mental health policy discussion held since the Carter administration, there were no decisions to be made. Tipper Gore and Bernard Arons made presentations, as did Richard Frank. The president asked some astute questions, reflecting his experience with mental health services from his days as governor of Arkansas. Nothing changed as a result of the meeting, but mental health clearly had a seat at the table in the crowded Roosevelt Room.

The failure of the health care reform process disappointed both participants as well as many citizens. Members of the Working Group on Mental Health and Substance Abuse shared the disappointment, but the process gave them a clear goal. The next step in the sequence of progressive iterations in mental health reform was to make "parity mental health benefits" a key tenet of federal mental health policy. The idea was to move from the staged approach offered at Tollgate 4 to full parity, as soon as possible. The process of moving in that direction began almost immediately.

Between 1994 and 1996 the main policy focus for advocates was on passage of a federal mental health parity act. This effort paralleled a process of developing parity legislation in states across the country. Beginning in 1971 with Connecticut, by 2004 as many as 34 states had enacted legislation mandating some level of insurance coverage for mental health services.[56] The earliest efforts, such as those in Connecticut and Massachusetts, required all insurers who offered insurance under the purview of state insurance regulation to offer some level of coverage for mental disorders. As time went on, these legislative initiatives fell under the rubric of "parity legislation," although in fact few extended comprehensive parity for all conditions to all insured citizens of a particular state. Some restricted the parity coverage to a limited list of conditions that were considered more severe and thus less subject to moral hazard. Others opened the benefits to cover all conditions but retained some limitations in services, such as a specified number of outpatient visits or inpatient days or higher co-payments for some services.[57] These state parity initiatives were a step in a more progressive direction, following the pattern of sequential reform, but they did not fully achieve their dual goal of improving insurance protection and ending a discriminatory practice. As long as some limitations remained, the goals were not achieved.

As managed behavioral health care became more common and more effective at controlling utilization and costs, opposition to parity tended to lessen in many states. If a parity initiative limited the expanded benefits to individuals who were receiving treatment within a managed care network of providers, it was easier to control costs; political opposition to parity initiatives eased as a result. Taken together, the evaluations of state parity indicated that parity was associated with some expansion of care and treatment, particularly outpatient services, while inpatient care contracted and costs remained fairly neutral. Managed care made parity possible, but not always palatable for providers and some service users, because of obstacles associated with utilization management and intrusion into the professional relationship by a third-party manager. Providers also resented the managed care companies' successful efforts to negotiate lower fees for their clinical services.[58]

Parity could achieve only limited objectives if it was to be implemented in a policy climate of resistance to "unfunded mandates" and fiscal austerity. The political requirement that parity be implemented with managed care meant that the goals of dramatically increasing access and quality with parity were less likely to be met. Furthermore, parity coverage did not include many of the rehabilitative and support services that the most impaired individuals required to maintain their recovery in the community. Lastly, parity did nothing to assist the 40-plus million individuals who had no health insurance. Advocates and policy supporters had to accept that (partial) parity would begin to improve insurance protection through reduced out-of-pocket expenses, easing the catastrophic financial effects of mental illness, and would move toward a less discriminatory and more inclusive policy.

State parity initiatives would have been the only needed policy instrument if federal legislation, called ERISA (Employee Retirement Income Security Act of 1974), had not given large employers who had employees in many states the right to self-insure and thus become exempt from state insurance regulations. Self-insured employer health plans, covering millions of Americans, were not required to follow the mandates of state parity laws. Federal legislation would be necessary if the effects of mental health parity were to be expanded to more citizens, particularly those in ERISA plans.

In 1992, even before health care reform began, Senators Pete Domenici (R-New Mexico) and Paul Wellstone (D-Minnesota) each responded to this problem by proposing a federal mental health parity law.[59] Each of these senators had personal experience with family members who had suffered from mental disorders. They, however, had somewhat different approaches to parity. In 1992 Senator Domenici favored a bill that would provide generous coverage for a limited number of the most severe mental disorders. Senator Wellstone sponsored a measure that would cover the full array of mental disorders, including substance use disorders. Neither bill was enacted, and health care reform preempted the issue for about a year. Once the reform effort failed, however, the two senators co-sponsored a bill that provided parity benefits for the treatment of all mental disorders except for those related to substance misuse. Their bill was debated in several sessions of Congress until 1996, when the bill was eventually scaled back.

What eventually became the Federal Mental Health Parity Act (PL 104-204) focused only on catastrophic insurance protection, in that it proposed parity with respect to annual and lifetime limits only. That is, according to the provisions of the law, any self-insured plan that offered mental health benefits could not have a higher annual or lifetime limit on insurance payments for mental illness than the limits that applied to other health conditions. Insurance benefits could still be otherwise curtailed for mental health treatment, and cost-sharing provisions could be higher for mental disorders than for other conditions. Other limitations were also added in that businesses with fewer than fifty employees were exempt from the parity policy, and any business that could show an expected increase in premium of more than 1 percent attributable to the mental health benefit could also be exempted from the parity law. Managed care was encouraged in order to assess the "medical necessity" of each episode of treatment. The Federal Mental Health Parity Act was passed in the summer of 1996 as a rider to the Veterans Affairs–Department of Housing and Urban Development appropriations bill. It went into effect in 1998 and had a sunset provision allowing the law to expire unless renewed at the end of 2001.

The GAO conducted a study that revealed implementation problems with the law.[60] It noted less than complete compliance with its provisions, and it found that half of firms that followed the law imposed additional limits on their mental health benefits. But the law, however limited, was viewed as another rhetorical victory for mental health advocacy. After all, it focused on the most important aspect of insurance limitations—catastrophic financial protection. From 1996 until his untimely death in a plane crash in 2000, Paul Wellstone and his unlikely partner on the other side of the aisle, Pete Domenici, worked to expand the scope of federal parity further. In spite of almost annual efforts to expand the Federal Mental Health Parity Act in Congress, as of this writing the law has been extended for a year without modification each time it was set to expire, beginning in 2001.

There had been earlier federal attempts to provide private health insurance parity benefits for the treatment of mental illnesses. The first federal effort to level the insurance playing field for individuals with mental disorders was undertaken by President Kennedy. As noted earlier, he directed the Civil Service Commission and its health insurance program for federal employees to offer the same insurance benefits for treating mental illnesses as for any other covered conditions. For more than a decade federal employees enjoyed generous mental health benefits.[61] After 1975, however, most plans began to restrict benefits. The High Option plan of Blue Cross/Blue Shield was the last federal plan to restrict mental health benefits, when in 1981 it was finally permitted to scale back its benefits after years of adverse selection. The Federal Employees Health Benefit (FEHB) Program had once been in the vanguard of progressive mental health benefits, but by the 1980s it reflected the insurance industry practice of placing limitations on mental health and substance abuse benefits.

Once again, however, the FEHB Program was to become a leader in progressive insurance reform in 2001, just as the Federal Mental Health Parity Act was getting ready to sunset.

Tipper Gore played an important role in setting the stage for further progress in federal mental health insurance reform and for advances in the profile of mental health more broadly. The strategy for change began in an unlikely venue—the Olympic Games in Atlanta in 1996.[62] While the wife of the vice president was attending a ceremony to release a report of the surgeon general on physical activity and health, she noted the considerable attention of the press and appreciated the opportunity to use an authoritative report to improve the health of the public. It occurred to her that a report of the surgeon general on mental health could have a similar beneficial effect. The surgeon general, after all, enjoyed great prestige, if not authority, when dealing with public health issues.

During the health care reform process, Tipper Gore's advocacy on behalf of mental health was often met with critical claims that mental health was a scientifically weak field. The most dismissive of the critics asserted that mental disorders were a myth—or, if not a myth, they were trivial or self-imposed problems. And some criticized the treatments as lacking in data to support their efficacy. Scientific reports by professional societies were considered self-serving; even reports from NIMH were dismissed as "advocacy." Tipper Gore thought that many of these criticisms could be answered by a scientific report on mental health from the surgeon general.

The following year Tipper Gore convinced Donna Shalala, secretary of DHHS, of the merits of her strategy. The secretary worked with the Office of the Surgeon General to begin the planning process for a report on mental health. In 1997 J. Jarrett Clinton was the acting surgeon general, filling the vacancy created by the resignation of the controversial Joycelyn Elders, the Arkansas physician appointed by President Clinton during his first administration.[63] Dr. Clinton approved the process for developing a mental health report and assigned lead responsibility to SAMHSA, with the process to be coordinated with the NIMH. Early in 1998 David Satcher, who had been director of the Centers for Disease Control and Prevention, was appointed surgeon general, and he embraced the mental health report with enthusiasm. The report was to review the science of mental health. It was not to be a policy document, and would be released in December 1999, before the start of the presidential campaign. Since the Gores were expected to be involved in that presidential campaign, it was important that the release of the surgeon general's mental health report not be seen as a political event.

Tipper Gore had another idea to advance the status and prestige of mental health, namely, a White House Conference on Mental Health. Held in June 1999, the FEHB Program again took center stage in federal mental health policy.[64] At the opening of the one-day conference President Clinton announced that he had directed the Office of Personnel Management, which operated the FEHB Program, to offer parity mental health and substance abuse benefits in all of its more than two hundred participating plans. The parity policy was to apply to providers within networks of clinicians and facilities that were associated with managed behavioral health care organizations. The Office of Personnel Management encouraged the plans to manage the care in a way that controlled the cost increases that were expected to accompany the expansion of benefits. The president called for a study to evaluate this policy experiment to guide policy in other health insurance programs considering parity. Given the difficulties in Congress associated with efforts to pass and then expand the Federal Mental Health Parity Act, this directive to the Office of Personnel Management represented a major shift in policy. Unlike previous parity policies, the new plan called for comprehensive mental health and substance abuse parity. The move was considered potentially quite influential, since the FEHB Program was the largest employer-based insurance program in the nation and covered more than 8 million individuals. The announcement of this change in the FEHB Program, alone, made the White House Conference on Mental Health a significant event in the history of federal mental health policy. Parity in the FEHB Program was set to commence January 1, 2001.

Released to the public in early December of 1999, *Mental Health—A Report of the Surgeon General* almost immediately accomplished its initial objective. It put mental health on the front page of the *New York Times.*[65] There was no real news in the report; the report itself was the news on an otherwise uneventful day. The report provided what Tipper Gore had envisioned. It was authoritative; its eight chapters with their three thousand citations delivered a review of the extensive scientific foundation of the mental health field. The report concluded that mental disorders were real health conditions, among the most disabling of them all; yet for almost every mental disorder there was a range of treatments whose efficacy had been established by research. The optimism associated with a choice of effective treatments (medications and psychotherapies) was tempered by the distressing finding that there was a substantial gap between research findings about therapies and what occurred in actual practice. Identifying this gap was the principal policy-relevant finding of the surgeon general's report.

The surgeon general himself spoke convincingly about his report. He knew its contents from beginning to end and promoted its basic ideas. He seemed fond of pointing out that "mental disorders *are* physical disorders," as if to say that the physical manifestations of these illnesses made them real—even to him. Satcher wanted to move public thinking away from the false dualism that separated the mind from body. He spoke of the research that demonstrated that the brain was changed in mental disorders and that it could be affected further by effective treatment, whether medication or psychotherapy. He became an important spokesperson for mental health and the need to close the gap between scientific findings and practice.

The report was not a consensus document in the sense that it was not produced by the deliberation of experts. In fact, there was only a Planning Board, a diverse group of stakeholders and experts, which met twice, and individual members participated as reviewers of the document, but did not vote on whether to accept its contents. They assisted the report's editors to think about the appropriate approach of each chapter, based on an outline and table of contents dictated by the charge from the Office of the Surgeon General and the DHHS. The table of contents followed a developmental framework with chapters on childhood and adolescence, adult life, and later life. There also were chapters on the organization and financing of the mental health services system and a chapter on the confidentiality of mental health information. The chapters themselves were divided into sections, and authors with expertise were commissioned to write papers according to the prescribed outline. Editors and science writers built the document from the various contributions, editing them as well as writing new sections and bridging materials. An executive group within DHHS reviewed the report and the comments of many reviewers. They assembled all of the criticism and decided with the senior scientific editor what to modify and how to proceed. Each of the operating divisions within DHHS eventually signed off on the document to indicate approval. The editors and writers had the freedom to present the findings "according to the best science," as Dr. Satcher was often heard to say.

Although the report was written with a minimum of controversy, several issues created tension during the writing process. All of the issues, however, were ultimately resolved. Initially it took some learning for SAMHSA and NIMH to collaborate. The senior NIH institute was uncomfortable at first with ceding a scientific review to the junior SAMHSA as lead organization. Over time the two organizations came to trust each other. In an effort to discredit the report, one reviewer during the review process leaked to the press the section of the report that discussed the effectiveness of electroconvulsive treatment. The section was clarified somewhat to reflect some differences in interpretation of the evidence on memory impairment following treatment, but the controversy quickly dissipated. In the end this issue did not disrupt the actual release of the report later in the year.

SAMHSA, the operating division with direct responsibility for the report, raised a more serious concern and was the last operating division to sign off on the report.

Officials in the agency expressed concern that the issues of culture, race, and ethnicity were not handled effectively in the draft report.[66] Various edits were proposed, and many were accepted, but there was some sentiment for developing a separate chapter on the subject. Another option gained more support and eventually prevailed, namely, the commissioning of a new report that would be a supplement and deal with culture, race, and ethnicity. It would have its own scientific editor and editorial review board. The result, *Mental Health: Culture, Race, and Ethnicity,* was released two years later in 2001.[67]

The only federal mental health policy issue to create any controversy was the section on managed behavioral health care.[68] Reviewer comments were evenly divided between those who felt that the chapter on organization and financing was too harsh in its reporting on managed care and those who felt it extolled it virtues inappropriately. Because the criticisms and comments were based more on opinion than on data, the section on managed care stood as originally written. Perhaps this was the only policy controversy because the report was explicitly not to be a policy document. Balancing that restriction with the wish to be policy-relevant was the greatest challenge for the report.

Julius Richmond provided the inspiration to find the right balance between a scientific report and a policy document. Richmond had been surgeon general and assistant secretary of DHEW during the Carter administration. He had been involved in Carter's PCMH, and had presided over the work group that prepared the National Plan. Early in the process of developing the report and on several occasions throughout the process, Richmond expressed concern that avoiding important policy issues was missing a once-in-a-lifetime opportunity. What emerged in the final report was a concluding chapter that identified eight courses of action that were implied by the foregoing review of the science of mental health and mental health services. The eight courses of action were the thinly veiled policy recommendations of a nonpolicy scientific document. These recommendations were of necessity broad if the report was to avoid becoming a policy document. They did, however, provide a framework that could be used in the future.

The policy recommendations were general in scope: first, the necessity of building the science base; second, the need to overcome stigma; third, the importance of improving public awareness of effective treatments; fourth, the adoption of measures to ensure an adequate supply of mental health services and providers; fifth, the importance of delivering state-of-the-art treatments; sixth, the need to tailor treatment to age, gender, race, and culture; seventh, the importance of facilitating entry into treatment; finally, the reduction of financial barriers to treatment.[69]

The document implicitly endorsed parity insurance coverage. "Equality between mental health coverage and other health coverage—a concept known as parity—is an affordable and effective objective," the report concluded. This conclusion, linked to a course of action, reinforced federal mental health policy activism on its many fronts. It endorsed the expansion of the Federal Mental Health Parity Act, and it supported President Clinton's directive to the Office of Personnel Management to implement parity benefits for federal employees.

In December 1999 the White House released the surgeon general's report with considerable fanfare and enthusiasm. Mental health advocates hoped that the landmark report would become the foundation for federal mental health policy in a Gore administration. But a few short weeks after federal employees began enjoying access to parity health insurance benefits in January 2001, another president was taking office. A George W. Bush and not an Al Gore administration would be responsible for translating the surgeon general's report into policy.

During the presidential campaign in 2000 George W. Bush promised that if he were elected, he would convene a commission on mental health services. This campaign promise did not attract much attention, not even among mental health advocates who viewed the proposal as part of the Bush campaign slogan promising a "compassionate conservatism." After the election the mental health commission turned out to be part of a specific "New Freedom Initiative" focused on improving community participation and integration for individuals who were disabled.[70] The New Freedom Initiative hoped to "tear down the barriers that face Americans with disabilities today."[71] It also addressed the Medicaid program and proposed some dramatic changes that would give states more flexibility in using this rapidly growing part of both state and federal budgets, but also might curtail entitlement to the program. The initiative was controversial; it called for a "transformation" rather than a "reform" of federal programs and policies. The New Freedom Commission on Mental Health was intended to make recommendations that would transform mental health services policy, because it was thought that the policy as it existed was too intractable for simple reform. Once convened, the commission remained true to this perception of the problem and to the intent to recommend a fundamental transformation.

Carter's PCMH had also pressed for fundamental change, but failed to accomplish its expansive objectives. Its success lay in making specific proposals that could be implemented incrementally in a sequence of policy moves. Such was the experience with the National Plan, and that experience was not lost on the President's New Freedom Commission on Mental Health.

The political challenge for the new commission was to build on previous experiences and reports, such as the National Plan and the surgeon general's report on mental health (both products of Democratic administrations), and to create something novel. The chances for success were limited by some elements of the charge of the new commission, but the process moved forward with some clever strategies designed to deal with these potential limitations.

President George W. Bush announced the President's New Freedom Commission on Mental Health in a speech in Albuquerque on April 29, 2002.[72] An executive order charged the commission "to conduct a comprehensive study of the United States mental health services delivery system . . . and make recommendations to the President." The commission was expected "to recommend improvements that allow adults with serious mental illness and children with severe emotional disturbance to live, work, learn, and participate fully in their communities." The cost of recommendations was expected to remain within current levels of spending. An interim report would be followed by the commission's final report within twelve months. "We need a health care system which treats mental illness with the same urgency as physical illness," noted the president in his Albuquerque speech. In so doing, he made clear that he supported health insurance parity for mental health treatment.

The executive order outlined five principles governing the work of the commission. First, the commission was to "focus on the desired outcomes of mental health care, which are to attain each individual's maximum level of employment, self-care, interpersonal relationships, and community participation." Second, the need was for "community-level models of care that efficiently coordinate the multiple health and human service providers and public and private payers involved in mental health treatment and delivery of services. Third, the commission should emphasize "those policies that maximize the utility of existing resources by increasing cost effectiveness and reducing unnecessary and burdensome regulatory barriers." Fourth, there was a need to determine ways in which mental health research findings could be used most effectively in influencing the delivery of services. Finally, the commission should "follow the principles of Federalism, and ensure that its recommendations promote innovation, flexibility and accountability at all levels of government and respect the constitutional role of the States and Indian tribes."[73] These principles guided the work of the commission, its final report, and the Action Agenda that followed the final report by two years.[74]

Michael Hogan, director of the Ohio Department of Mental Health and a widely respected leader in mental health services for several decades, was appointed chair of the President's New Freedom Commission on Mental Health. Claire Heffernan, a lawyer who had served on the staff of Senator Kit Bond (R-Missouri), was appointed executive director, and H. Stanley Eichenauer, a social worker and mental health administrator, became the deputy executive director. The fourteen nonfederal commissioners formed a diverse group; most were local mental health experts, more than a few from Texas or personal acquaintances of the president. Seven additional commissioners represented federal agencies, including SAMHSA, NIMH, the Department of Veterans Affairs, the Department of Labor, the Department of Education, the Department of Housing and Urban Development, and the Centers for Medicare and Medicaid.

Although it had been nearly a quarter of a century since the PCMH, there were several similarities between the two commissions and some lessons to be heeded.[75] First, fragmentation of mental health services and policies was a central problem at both points in time. The difference, noted Hogan, reflected the fact that the research evidence had led to the conclusion "that systems integration is not the answer."[76] Second, both commissions were expected to recommend far-reaching changes—"transformation" was the term used by the Bush administration—yet the lesson of the PCMH was that fundamental change was elusive, but small sequential steps guided by a specific set of recommendations were more likely to bear fruit. Third, both commissions were required to review the science of mental health and mental health services as the basis for their work. Thus the New Freedom Commission could rely on the recently completed report of the surgeon general, which would be its scientific foundation.

Hogan was very aware of these lessons and implemented several strategies to improve the likely outcome of the commission's work. He made available to all of the commissioners a report on the "quiet success" of the National Plan in order to encourage them to think about making specific incremental recommendations. To further that objective he and Heffernan organized the commissioners into sixteen subcommittees. Each subcommittee was expected to prepare a report and a set of recommendations in its area; each was given access to resources to hire a consultant to write a paper to assist in preparing that subcommittee report. The recommendations of the final report of the commission would be drawn from these subcommittee reports, but only one or two from each. Uncertain that the White House would accept some of the more ambitious recommendations, Hogan and the commissioners hoped that their subcommittee reports and recommendations would become part of the record of their work and serve in a role similar to that of the National Plan. The interim report was designed as a dramatic critique of the system of care, raising the stakes for the work of the commission and the response of the White House and the nation. The final report would contain the most important recommendations and their rationale, but the subcommittee reports might prove as important as the final report itself.

Hogan also positioned the surgeon general's report on mental health as the scientific basis for the commission's work. It would not have been possible to conduct a comprehensive review of all of mental health and mental health services in the one year allotted for its work. It was therefore convenient to rely on the surgeon general's report. The recommended courses of action from that report were aligned with the executive order and were reflected in the deliberations of the commission.

Six months after it had begun its work, the commission released its Interim Report.[77] It was a scathing indictment of the mental health service system. The report identified a number of major barriers to mental health care. There were both fragmentation and gaps in care for children with severe emotional disturbances and for adults with serious mental disorders. High unemployment and disability were characteristic among adults with severe mental illness. Older adults with mental disorders were not receiving care. Finally, mental health and suicide prevention were not yet national priorities. These barriers served as the rationale for the commission's reports and recommendations.

Recovery from mental illness was a strong, recurring theme in the commission's discussions. The surgeon general's report on mental health had presented evidence that the long-term outcomes for individuals with some of the most severe mental disorders were better than previously believed. Research provided a reason for optimism about the prospects for recovery. For many, recovery meant participating fully in life in the community—the very words in the executive order that created the president's New Freedom Commission. For others it meant hope and possibilities for a more normal life in spite of continued impairments. The importance of the vision of recovery was underscored at a meeting of the commission with Rosalynn Carter.[78] She observed that the idea that recovery was possible—even expected—was the most striking contrast between the thinking about mental illnesses at the time of the Bush Commission and the ideas about mental illnesses at the time of the PCMH.

The final report was released on July 22, 2003. Once again the commission criticized the mental health service delivery system as fragmented and disorganized, requiring no less than a "fundamental transformation of the Nation's approach to mental health care." Entitled *Achieving the Promise: Transforming Mental Health Care in America*, it outlined six goals for a transformed mental health system: first, that mental health was essential to overall health; second, that mental health care had to be consumer and family driven; third, that disparities in mental health care had to be eliminated; fourth, that early mental health screening, assessment, and referral to services had to become common practice; fifth, to ensure that excellent mental health care was delivered and research accelerated; finally, that technology be employed to access mental health care and information. "We envision a future," the report noted, "when everyone with a mental illness will recover, a future when mental illnesses can be prevented or cured, a future when everyone with a mental illness at any stage of life has access to effective treatment and supports—essentials for living, working, learning, and participating fully in the community."[79]

The goals were further subdivided into nineteen specific recommendations. Few if any of these recommendations were specific or could be linked immediately to federal mental health policy or national leadership for other levels of government or the private sector. More work was required if these goals and recommendations were to be transformed into real policies and programs. The commission followed the lead of the White House and did not present anything more specific than these general recommendations—in many cases hardly more specific than the recommended actions in the surgeon general's report.

In the Bush administration budgets were tight. Federal mental health policy occupied an extremely low priority for the administration, which had become embroiled in foreign wars, Medicare modernization, a Medicaid spending crisis, and plans to transform the Social Security system. SAMHSA was given lead responsibility to develop an action agenda that would make more specific recommendations. SAMHSA also planned to release the subcommittee reports with their more detailed recommendations. A group of federal agencies met regularly to consider ways in which they could better collaborate on mental health issues and in which they could align their policies with the recommendations of the commission. The Department of Veterans Affairs made notable progress in that regard, but little occurred outside of the government.

In 2002 mental health advocates organized themselves into a Campaign for Mental Health Reform to try to speak with one voice and press for implementation of the recommendations of the commission. [80] At first the campaign involved four major mental health advocacy organizations—the National Mental Health Association, the National Alliance for the Mentally Ill, the Bazelon Center for Mental Health Law, and the National Association of State Mental Health Program Directors. Later it added a dozen other advocacy and professional organizations. A year went by with repeated promises of an Action Agenda, but none was forthcoming. Five of the subcommittee reports were issued by SAMHSA, but not all of them appeared in the two years following the release of *Achieving the Promise*. The campaign decided to begin work on its own action agenda and set of specific recommendations.

Federal mental health policy occupied such a low priority that even the centerpiece of advocacy—comprehensive mental health parity in health insurance coverage—was not moving along a path toward legislation. The Federal Mental Health Parity Act was once again extended without modification at the end of 2005. Why was there no progress on parity? The surgeon general had supported both its correctness and its feasibility. President Clinton had made sure at the White House Conference on Mental Health that federal employees, including members of Congress, would have parity. Even President George W. Bush affirmed his support for parity. But there was no comprehensive federal parity law and Medicare continued to retain a discriminatory mental health benefit.

The lessons of the National Plan and the sequential implementation of federal mental health policy had made clear the need for a blueprint or roadmap to follow toward reform. Presidential commissions might call for a "bold new approach" and "transformation," but without a national plan or an action agenda, meaningful, progressive change was unlikely. By the end of July 2005 a confluence of events gave a new boost of hope that federal mental health policy might move forward on the heels of all this effort:

Late in May the DHHS put the results of the Evaluation of Mental Health and Substance Abuse Insurance Parity in the FEHB Program on its Website. The study had concluded that parity was implemented as intended in the context of managed care. It had ended a discriminatory policy and improved insurance protection by reducing out-of-pocket payments for individuals who were treated for mental and addictive disorders. It had done so without adverse increases in total spending or decreases in quality.[81] Congress would be able to use these findings in its deliberations over the Federal Mental Health Parity Act in the upcoming session of Congress.

In July SAMHSA finally released the federal Action Agenda, two years after the final report of the commission. Entitled *Transforming Mental Health Care in America*, the agenda was the result of the work of six cabinet-level departments—Education, DHHS, HUD, Justice, Labor, Veterans Affairs, and SSA.[82] The report followed the five principles from the original executive order and offered seventy specific steps. Its commitments included the implementation of the National Strategy for Suicide Prevention, grants to promote organizational transformation of state mental health authorities, the expansion of the implementation of evidence-based practices, the design of an electronic medical record for mental health services, and the improvement of the service system for children with mental health problems. No specific resources were detailed; although some of these recommendations could be funded from existing agency budgets, others would require additional appropriations. As was the case with the National Plan during the decade of the 1980's, it would take time to see if the action agenda produced incremental results.

A week after the release of the federal Action Agenda, the Campaign for Mental Health Reform issued *Emergency Response: A Roadmap for Federal Action in America's Mental Health Crisis.* [83] The campaign's roadmap contained twenty-eight action items. One focused on diverting people with a mental illness from the criminal justice system and another called for an end to "warehousing" children in institutions. Several of the action steps focused on specific financing policy issues in Medicaid and in SSI. In many ways the steps resembled the recommendations in the National Plan from which the idea of the roadmap derives. The campaign once again explicitly called for parity—for an end to discrimination in private health insurance plans and in Medicare.

The themes of federal mental health policy in 2005 in some ways are similar to those of 1995 and 1980. Fragmentation in policies and practices had to be replaced with coordination and alignment of finances with the needs of individuals with mental disorders. Policies and practices should provide the right incentives to deliver effective treatments and supports. And policies should be fair and equitable and recognize the right of individuals with mental disorders to live full lives in their communities.

A sequence of incremental steps may lead federal mental health policy in a direction that addresses these themes and concerns. History suggests that the roadmaps and action agendas can guide the way. Nevertheless, preoccupation with other problems and a thrust to diminish federal social welfare responsibilities also have the potential to threaten the well-being of persons with serious mental disorders and disabilities. Only time will tell whether the American people and their elected representatives have the will to deal with the needs of a severely disabled population encouraged by the prospect of recovery.

Epilogue

Much has been accomplished in mental health policy, but much remains to be achieved. Recently two economists, Richard Frank and Sherry Glied have argued that during the past half century the mental health and well-being of Americans have improved. The fate of those who are poorest and most impaired, however, has deteriorated. Frank and Glied conclude that with respect to our mental health we are better, but not well.[1]

Our analysis of the history of federal mental health policy over the same period finds that this mix of progress and disappointment derives from the interplay of the work of policy realists and policy idealists. Policy realists have taken advantage of opportunities for incremental change within the realities of an essentially conservative political process. Policy idealists, by contrast, have set out a vision of fundamental change that, though never actually achieved, has served as an objective—a goal or target for those who influence or move the levers of change. A series of presidential commissions and high-level reports have offered a blueprint or roadmap for progress. Policy idealists have been disappointed that their lofty objectives have not yet been achieved, while policy realists have taken opportunities for incremental advances along a sequence of small progressive changes. Together they have taken strategic opportunities to move forward on a set of federal policies for individuals who experience a mental disorder—or for any one of us who might experience a mental illness.

The differing worldviews of realists and idealists have created a constructive tension in federal mental health policy. In truth, some advocates and policymakers hold aspects of both worldviews at the same time. The resolution of the tension has resulted in progress when the vision of the idealists has been coupled with the creative and strategic activities of the realists, who take advantage of political opportunities to produce change.

We have examined the period from the end of World War II to the present time. Our analysis began with the rise of the community mental health reforms in the first half of this fifty-year history and continued with the community support reform of the second half of that period. We have also written about contemporary events. In many instances we have been influenced by and even participated in these events. The closeness in time and place is a challenge to objectivity, and the time frame makes it even more difficult to draw conclusions. The impact of many of the events and processes has yet to be realized in terms of specific changes and longer-term effects.

The Joint Commission on Mental Illness and Health began as an initiative to advance incremental changes in care in mental hospitals, although in the end it offered a variety of broad, if unfocused, demands. Its proposals did not, however, alter in fundamental ways the existing institutional policy. At the same time Robert H. Felix and his NIMH colleagues were developing a radical alternative, the creation of community mental health centers (CMHCs) that would have no relationship to public mental hospitals. Indeed, they saw the CMHC as an institution that within a generation would replace institutional care. Creating a CMHC program not only established a new, fundamental reform that changed the locus of mental health services, but also transferred mental health policy leadership from the states to the federal government. CMHCs, at least in theory, were designed to provide an array of services to individuals with mental disorders. In addition to serving some individuals with severe conditions, their mission was expanded to treat individuals with a broad range of conditions. This drift away from the most impaired established a new set of expectations but also produced a counter-reaction of concern about abandonment of individuals with disabling conditions who fared poorly in the communities where they now lived under the new policy of deinstitutionalization. In the mid-1970s the federal government was charged to "do more" by the General Accounting Office, an instruction that once again set reform in motion.

The problems of the CMHC program in the late 1970s paralleled the appearance of new policies designed to share power between the federal government and the states. They also gave rise to another fundamental reform in mental health services, the community support movement. This movement redefined the challenge of severe and persistent mental disorders as a broad social problem requiring an array of services extending far beyond the reach of traditional health and mental health services and traditional health care institutions. The NIMH Community Support Program was a federal grant initiative directed both at local communities and at state mental health authorities.

Like the Joint Commission two decades before, the President's Commission on Mental Health in 1977 began with a more limited set of objectives that grew as its work continued. Its goals extended beyond concerns about individuals who already experienced a mental illness to those who might develop a mental disorder and to a broad set of objectives for social change and societal betterment. The commission report encompassed prevention and mental health promotion, mental health awareness and public education, as well as care and treatment. It led to two important and very different sets of policy actions.

One policy initiative—the Mental Health Systems Act—was a radical piece of legislation that altered the relationship between the stewards of mental health policy in the federal government (the NIMH) and state mental health authorities. It expanded community-based mental health services along a model of community support and focused attention primarily on individuals with disabling mental disorders. The Mental Health Systems Act addressed traditional categorical mental health resources, allocated exclusively for mental health treatment and outside the mainstream funding mechanisms that financed the rest of health care.

The second policy initiative was the National Plan for the Chronically Mentally Ill. It was a grab bag of incremental changes in the mainstream social and health care programs upon which individuals with severe and persistent mentally ill persons had come to depend while living outside of institutional settings in their communities. When Reagan defeated Carter in 1980, the radical if unfocused reforms of the Mental Health Systems Act were reversed. Nevertheless, the National Plan provided a blueprint for a sequence of progressive incremental changes throughout the decade.

The Clinton health care reform effort was a failed effort at fundamental change in the 1990s. The effort included considerations of mental health and substance abuse in its deliberations and its legislative proposals. The changes, however, were considered to be too radical to be implemented and the initiative went down to defeat. Paradoxically, the initiative was a rhetorical victory for mental health policy. It led to an incremental change in mental health financing—the Federal Mental Health Parity Act—paralleling insurance parity legislation in the states. The 1990s also saw a series of other small gains in federal recognition for mental health, embodied in a White House Conference on Mental Health, a report from the surgeon general on mental health, several action papers and supplements to the report, and mental health and substance abuse insurance parity for federal employees.

Fulfilling a campaign promise, President George W. Bush announced that he was creating a President's New Freedom Commission on Mental Health in 2002. The executive order establishing the commission had limited boundaries but also reflected a wish for "transformation." The commission struggled with the tensions of encouraging transformation and promoting full participation in the community while coping with a mandate for limited resources and a focus only on adults with severe mental disorders and children with serious emotional disturbances. As did the members of the JCMIH and the PCMH, commission members broadened their recommendations beyond their charge. They called for insurance parity and for advancing research in order to find a cure for mental disorders. They also pushed for programs that would exceed the then-current levels of expenditure that were set as a ceiling in the executive order. Behind the main recommendations in *Achieving the Promise,* the commission's final report in 2003, were fifteen issue papers, that made even broader recommendations. Some of the issue papers were published and others remained unpublished but available underground, as the National Plan on the Chronically Mentally Ill had been in the 1980s. In 2005 a federal action agenda introduced some new programs, but there was no new funding to support real transformation. At almost the same time Coalition for Mental Health Reform also issued a "roadmap for federal action."

Much remains to be accomplished in terms of implementing these recommendations. The next decade will tell us whether transformation will mean radical or incremental change or simply remain as a political slogan. It is difficult to see how fundamental change can result with so little change in the resource base and an adherence to the rules for applying mainstream programs to the special problems of individuals with severe and persistent mental disorders. The impact of these new initiatives may be measured once again in terms of incremental changes in specific programs. Will a comprehensive, federal insurance parity law be passed? Will states transform their mental health systems, pooling resources across the many state agencies that affect individuals with mental illness? Will new evidence-based service programs be implemented? Will Medicaid continue to finance the mental health system? Will new treatments be covered in the Medicaid of the future? Will people with mental illnesses on the disability rolls return to work? Will they be able to live in decent housing in their neighborhoods? We hope that they will fulfill the objectives of the President's New Freedom Commission on Mental Health—"to live, work, learn, and participate fully in their communities."[2]

Beneath these important questions lies an even more fundamental ethical and moral issue, the question of society's obligation toward individuals whose disability from a severe and persistent mental disorder creates partial or full dependency. It has often been noted that a society will be judged by the manner in which it treats its most vulnerable and dependent citizens. In this sense persons with severe mental disorders have a moral claim upon society's compassion and above all, upon its material assistance. Many of these persons also have a strong wish to participate in their care and in making mental health policy. The new interest in recovery and self-directed care means that individuals with severe and persistent mental disorders expect more of themselves, as well, and they seek respect as full partners in the process of improving services and resources to support recovery and transformation.

Notes

Prologue

1. Larry D. Eldridge, "'Crazy Brained': Mental Illness in Colonial America," *Bulletin of the History of Medicine* 70 (1996): 361–386; Gerald N. Grob, *Mental Institutions in America: Social Policy to 1875* (New York: Free Press, 1973), chap. 1; Mary A. Jimenez, *Changing Faces of Madness: Early American Attitudes and Treatment of the Insane* (Hanover, N.H.: University Press of New England, 1987), passim.

2. Dorothea L. Dix, *Memorial to the Legislature of Massachusetts, 1843* (Boston: Munroe & Francis, 1843), 4; *Memorial Soliciting a State Hospital for the Insane Submitted to the Legislature of New Jersey, January 23, 1845* (Trenton, N.J.: n.p., 1845), 3; *Memorial Soliciting Enlarged and Improved Accommodations for the Insane of the State of Tennessee* (Nashville: B. R. M'Kennie, 1847), 1–2.

3. Dora L. Costa, *The Evolution of Retirement: An American Economic History, 1880–1980* (Chicago: University of Chicago Press, 1998), 184–185.

4. U.S. Bureau of the Census, *Patients in Mental Institutions 1940* (Washington, D.C.: Government Printing Office, 1943), 63.

5. Joseph Zubin and Grace C. Scholz, *Regional Differences in the Hospitalization and Care of Patients with Mental Disease*, Public Health Reports, Supplement no. 159 (Washington, D.C.: Government Printing Office, 1940), 74.

6. Gerald N. Grob, *The State and the Mentally Ill: A History of Worcester State Hospital in Massachusetts, 1830–1920* (Chapel Hill: University of North Carolina Press, 1966), 87–90; Grob, *Mental Institutions*, 194–197.

7. Worcester State Lunatic Hospital, *Annual Report*, 30 (1862): 18ff.

8. Grob, *Mental Institutions*, chapter 7; Grob, *Mental Illness and American Society, 1875–1940* (Princeton: Princeton University Press, 1983), chap. 4.

9. Grob, *Mental Illness and American Society*, chaps. 4, 7; Grob, *The State and the Mentally Ill*, 331–332.

10. Grob, *Mental Illness and American Society*, 91–92.

11. U.S. Bureau of the Census, *Insane and Feeble-Minded in Hospitals and Institutions 1904* (Washington, D.C.: Government Printing Office, 1906), 37; U.S. Bureau of the Census, *Insane and Feeble-Minded in Institutions 1910* (Washington, D.C.: Government Printing Office, 1914), 59; U.S. Bureau of the Census, *Patients in Hospitals for Mental Disease 1923* (Washington, D.C.: Government Printing Office, 1926), 36.

12. Neil A. Dayton, *New Facts on Mental Disorders: Study of 89,190 Cases* (Springfield, Ill.: Charles C. Thomas, 1940), 414–438.

13. American Psychiatric Association, *Report on Patients over 65 in Public Mental Hospitals* (Washington, D.C.: American Psychiatric Association, 1960).

14. Morton Kramer, H. Goldstein, R. H. Israel, and N. A. Johnson, *A Historical Study of the Disposition of First Admissions to a State Mental Hospital: Experience of Warren State Hospital during the Period 1916–1950*, U.S. Public Health Service Publication no. 445 (1955), and the same authors' "Application of Life Table Methodology to the Study of Mental Hospital Populations," in American Psychiatric Association, *Psychiatric Research Report* 5 (1956): 49–87.

15. See Elizabeth Lunbeck, *The Psychiatric Persuasion: Knowledge, Gender, and Power in Modern America* (Princeton: Princeton University Press, 1994).

16. Thomas W. Salmon, "Some New Fields in Neurology and Psychiatry," *Journal of Nervous and Mental Disease* 46 (1917): 90–99. The history of the mental hygiene movement can be followed in Grob, *Mental Illness and American Society*, 144–178; Norman Dain, *Clifford W. Beers: Advocate for the Insane* (Pittsburgh: University of Pittsburgh Press, 1980); Margo Horn, *Before It's Too Late: The Child Guidance Movement in the United States, 1922–1945* (Philadelphia: Temple University Press, 1989); and Theresa R. Richardson, *The Century of the Child: The Mental Hygiene Movement and Social Policy in the United States and Canada* (Albany: State University of New York Press, 1989).

17. Lothar B. Kalinowsky and Paul H. Hoch, *Shock Treatments and Other Somatic Procedures in Psychiatry* (New York: Grune & Stratton, 1946), 243. See also Jack D. Pressman, *Last Resort: Psychosurgery and the Limits of Medicine* (New York: Oxford University Press, 1998).

18. In this volume we will in general deal neither with the history of federal policy in regard to children's mental health nor with the Veterans Administration, which also occupies a significant niche in federal general and mental health policy. The history of the VA—as yet unwritten—deserves a volume in its own right.

Chapter 1 — Winds of Change

1. The term *patient care episode* represents the sum of two numbers: residents at the beginning of the year or on the active role of outpatient facilities; and admissions during the year. The first is an unduplicated count; the second includes duplications, since some individuals had multiple admissions.

2. Raymond G. Fuller, "A Study of the Administration of State Psychiatric Services," *Mental Hygiene* 38 (1954): 181–182. Data on psychiatrists compiled from *List of Fellows and Members of the American Psychiatric Association 1940* (n.p., 1942).

3. Joanne E. Atay and Ronald W. Manderscheid, *Additions and Resident Patients at End of Year, State and County Mental Hospitals . . . 2001* (Rockville, Md.: Center for Mental Health Services, 2003), viii.

4. The struggle within the American Psychiatric Association can be followed in Gerald N. Grob, *From Asylum to Community: Mental Health Policy in Modern America* (Princeton: Princeton University Press, 1991), esp. 24–43.

5. Robert H. Felix, "Mental Public Health: A Blueprint," presentation at St. Elizabeths Hospital, April 21, 1945, Felix Papers, National Library of Medicine (NLM), Bethesda, Md.; Felix and R. V. Bowers, "Mental Hygiene and Socio-Environmental Factors," *Milbank Memorial Fund Quarterly* 26 (1948): 125–147.

6. Albert Deutsch, *The Shame of the States* (New York: Harcourt, Brace, 1948); Albert Q. Maisel, "Bedlam 1946," *Life* 20 (May 6, 1946): 102–118; Mike Gorman, "Oklahoma Attacks Its Snakepits," *Reader's Digest* 53 (September 1948): 139–160; Mary Jane Ward, *The Snake Pit* (New York: Random House, 1946), serialized in the *Reader's Digest* 48 (May 1948): 129–168. A fuller account can be found in Grob, *From Asylum to Community*, and esp. 72–76.

7. Data on the location of psychiatrists is taken from the following: *Biographical Directory of Fellows & Members of the American Psychiatric Association as of October 1, 1957* (New York: R. R. Bowker, 1958); "Distribution of Members of the American Psychiatric Association, 1910–1960," Miscellaneous Papers, Box 1, Archives of the

APA, Washington, D.C.; Joint Information Service of the APA, Fact Sheet no. 2, May 1957, and no. 10, August 1959; David A. Boyd, "Current and Future Trends in Psychiatric Residency Training," *Journal of Medical Education* 33 (1958): 345–346.

8. Harry C. Solomon, "The American Psychiatric Association in Relation to American Psychiatry," *American Journal of Psychiatry* 115 (1958): 1–9; *New York Times,* May 13, 1958, 31, May 16, 23; Robert C. Hunt to Solomon, June 17, 1958, Solomon to Hunt, June 19, 1958, Solomon Papers, APA Archives; Robert C. Hunt, "The State Hospital Stereotype," statement before the APA Commission on Long Term Planning, October 30, 1959, Records of the Medical Director's Office, 200–211, APA Archives.

9. President's Scientific Research Board, *Science and Public Policy,* 5 vols. (Washington, D.C.: Government Printing Office, 1947), 1:3, 113–118.

10. Gerald N. Grob, *Mental Illness and American Society, 1875–1940* (Princeton: Princeton University Press, 1983), 308–315.

11. Franklin G. Ebaugh, *The Care of the Psychiatric Patient in General Hospitals* (Chicago: American Hospital Association, 1940).

12. Robert H. Felix interview by Dr. Jeanne Brand, April 2, 1964, W.D. Miles Oral History Collection, History of Medicine Division, NLM; Felix interview by Daniel Blain, Blain Papers, Box 24, Folder 7, APA Archives; Felix interview by Milton J. E. Senn, March 8, 1979, Senn Collection, OH76, NLM; Alanson W. Willcox to Felix, February 20, 1945 (with draft bill), Mary E. Switzer Papers, Schlesinger Library, Radcliffe College, Cambridge, Mass.; Mary Switzer interview, 1966, OH161, APA Archives; Mary E. Switzer to Karl A. Menninger, March 14, 1945, Switzer File, Menninger Foundation Papers, Kansas Historical Society, Topeka, Kans.; 79-1 Congress, *National Neuropsychiatric Institute Act: Hearing before a Subcommittee of the Committee on Interstate and Foreign Commerce, House of Representatives . . . 1945* (Washington, D.C.: Government Printing Office, 1945); 79-2 Congress, *National Neuropsychiatric Institute Act: Hearings before a Subcommittee of the Committee on Education and Labor, United States Senate . . . 1946* (Washington, D.C.: Government Printing Office, 1946).

13. Chap. 538, *U.S. Statutes at Large,* 60 (1946): 421–426; Felix interview by Blain.

14. Robert H. Felix, "Mental Disorders as a Public Health Problem," *American Journal of Psychiatry* 106 (1949): 401–406; Paul V. Lemkau, *Mental Hygiene in Public Health* (New York: McGraw-Hill, 1949).

15. 80-2 Congress, *Hearings before the Subcommittee of the Committee on Appropriations House of Representatives . . . on the Department of Labor-Federal Security Agency Appropriation Bill for 1949* (Washington, D.C.: Government Printing Office, 1948), part 2, 271–287.

16. Felix and Bowers, "Mental Hygiene and Socio-Environmental Factors," 125–147; Felix, "Mental Public Health," passim; Felix, "Mental Disorders as a Public Health Problem," 401–406.

17. Felix interview by Brand.

18. PHS Mental Hygiene Division, "Annual Report for Fiscal Year 1947," 5–6, typed copy in NIMH Records, Subject Files, 1940–1951, Box 82, Record Group 511.2, National Archives (NA), Washington, D.C.; Robert H. Felix, "The Relation of the National Mental Health Act to State Health Authorities," *Public Health Reports* 62 (1947): 46–47; Felix, "The National Mental Health Program—A Progress Report," ibid., 63 (1948): 837–839. I (GNG) examined the NIMH records when they were still at the Washington National Record Center, Suitland, Md.

19. Lawrence J. Friedman, *Menninger: The Family and the Clinic* (New York: Knopf, 1990), 170–180, 194–197; J. Sanbourne Bockoven, *Moral Treatment in Community Mental Health* (New York: Springer Publishing Co., 1972), 114–146.

20. Maxwell Jones, *The Therapeutic Community: A New Treatment Method in Psychiatry* (New York: Basic Books, 1953); Alfred H. Stanton and Morris S. Schwartz, *The Mental Hospital: A Study of Institutional Participation in Psychiatric Illness and Treatment* (New York: Basic Books, 1954); Milton Greenblatt, Richard H. York, Esther L. Brown, and Robert W. Hyde, *From Custodial to Therapeutic Patient Care in Mental Hospitals* (New York: Russell Sage Foundation, 1955); Robert N. Rapoport, *Community as Doctor* (Springfield, Ill.: Charles C. Thomas, 1960).

21. Council of State Governments, *The Mental Health Programs of the Forty-Eight States: A Report to the Governors' Conference* (Chicago: Council of State Governments, 1950); Milbank Memorial Fund, *The Elements of a Community Mental Health Program* (New York: Milbank Memorial Fund, 1956), and *Programs for Community Mental Health* (New York: Milbank Memorial Fund, 1957).

22. The development of psychopharmacological agents can be followed in Judith P. Swazey, *Chlorpromazine in Psychiatry: A Study of Therapeutic Innovation* (Cambridge: MIT Press, 1974), and David Healy, *The Creation of Psychopharmacology* (Cambridge: Harvard University Press, 2002).

23. "Gains in Outpatient Psychiatric Services, 1959," *Public Health Reports* 75 (1960): 1092–1094; Vivian B. Norman, Beatrice M. Rosen, and Anita K. Bahn, "Psychiatric Outpatient Clinics in the United States, 1959," *Mental Hygiene* 46 (1962): 321–343.

24. National Advisory Mental Health Council, Minutes of Meeting, December 11–12, 1950, 11–14, March 9–11, 1955, 5–7, Record Group 90, NA; NIMH, *Evaluation in Mental Health . . . Report of the Subcommittee on Evaluation of Mental Health Activities, Community Services Committee, National Advisory Mental Health Council*, U.S. Public Health Service Publication 413 (1955), 1, 3, 57.

25. Harold Sampson, D. Ross, B. Engle, and F. Livson, *A Study of Suitability for Outpatient Clinic Treatment of State Mental Hospital Admissions*, California Department of Mental Hygiene, Research Report no. 1 (1957). A briefer version appeared under the title "Feasibility of Community Clinic Treatment for State Mental Hospital Patients," *Archives of Neurology and Psychiatry* 80 (1958): 71–77.

26. See Morton Kramer, *Some Implications of Trends in the Usage of Psychiatric Facilities for Community Mental Health Programs and Related Research*, U.S. Public Health Service Publication 1434 (Washington, D.C.: Government Printing Office, 1967); Kramer, "Epidemiology, Biostatistics, and Mental Health Planning," in American Psychiatric Association, *Psychiatric Research Reports* 22 (1967): 1–68; Kramer, C. Taube, and S. Starr, "Patterns of Use of Psychiatric Facilities by the Aged: Current Status, Trends, and Implications," ibid., 23 (1968): 89–150.

27. See Thomas N. Bonner, *Iconoclast: Abraham Flexner and a Life in Learning* (Baltimore: Johns Hopkins University Press, 2002).

28. For a detailed history of the JCMIH, see Grob, *From Asylum to Community*, 181–208.

29. Although the original mandate of the JCMIH was to study both mental illness and mental retardation, the latter was deleted from the agenda relatively early. The care and treatment of the latter was of marginal concern to most psychiatrists, and by the 1950s there was clear evidence of friction between mainstream psychiatrists and those concerned with retardation.

30. Minutes of the Organizational Meeting of the Board of Trustees, September 11, 1955, Box 5, JCMIH Papers, APA Archives.

31. The published monographs included Rashi Fein, *Economics of Mental Illness* (New York: Basic Books, 1958); Marie Jahoda, *Current Concepts of Positive Mental Health* (New York: Basic Books, 1958); George W. Albee, *Mental Health Manpower Trends* (New York: Basic Books, 1959); Gerald Gurin, J. Veroff, and S. Field, *Americans View Their Mental Health* (New York: Basic Books, 1960); Reginald Robinson, D. F. DeMarche, and M. K. Wagle, *Community Resources in Mental Health* (New York: Basic Books, 1960); Wesley Allinsmith and G. W. Goethals, *The Role of the Schools in Mental Health* (New York: Basic Books, 1962); Richard B. McCann, *The Churches and Mental Health* (New York: Basic Books, 1962); Richard J. Plunkett and John E. Gordon, *Epidemiology and Mental Illness* (New York: Basic Books, 1960); and Morris S. Schwartz, C. G. Schwartz, and M. G. Field, *Social Approaches to Mental Patient Care* (New York: Columbia University Press, 1964). William F. Soskin's report on research resources in mental health was never published.

32. "The Joint Commission on Mental Illness and Health, Inc. . . . Boston . . . August 20–21, 1960" (typed stenographic transcript), 105–147, 158–171, Box 2, JCMIH Papers.

33. *Action for Mental Health: Final Report of the Joint Commission on Mental Illness and Health 1961* (New York: Basic Books, 1961), 22–23.

34. Ibid., 8, 26–85.

35. Ibid., 213–241.

36. Ibid., 241–260.

37. Ibid., 260–268.

38. Ibid., 267–275.

39. Ibid., 275–295.

40. Ibid., 330–331.

41. JCMIH Press Release, March 24, 1961, in R. L. Robinson File *Action for Mental Health,* Box 6, JCMIH Papers.

42. For a detailed discussion of the reaction of the APA to *Action for Mental Health,* see Grob, *From Asylum to Community,* 210–213. The final judgment of the organization can be found in Memo by Walter Barton, with revised draft of APA Council statement, December 22, 1961, JCMIH Papers; APA Executive Committee Minutes, January 15, 1962, 4–6, APA Board of Trustee Papers, APA Archives; APA Council, "A Position Statement with Interpretive Commentary and Commendations," *Mental Hospitals,* 13 (1962): 68–69, 72.

43. Grob, *From Asylum to Community,* 213–216.

44. *Planning of Facilities for Mental Health Services: Report of the Surgeon General's Ad Hoc Committee on Planning for Mental Health Facilities,* Public Health Service Publication 8087 (1961), ii–v, 2–5, 25–34; *State Government* 35 (1962): 2–19.

45. Robert H. Felix Interview, August 5, 1964 (OH120), APA Archives; Felix, "Implications and Implementation of the Joint Commission Report at the Federal Level," speech at the Governors' Conference, November 1961, Felix Papers; Philip Sapir to Felix, October 23, 1959; Richard H. Williams to Felix, October 22, 1959; Felix to John R. Seeley, January 22, 1959, NIMH Records, Mental Health Subject Files 1957–1960, Box 7, Record Group 511.2.

46. Grob, *From Asylum to Community,* 219–220.

47. John F. Kennedy to Abraham Ribicoff, December 1, 1961, White House Central Files, Box 338, Folder HE 1-1, John F. Kennedy Library, Boston; Henry A. Foley, *Community Mental Health Legislation: The Formative Process* (Lexington, Mass.: Lexington Books, 1975), 33–37.

48. "National Institute of Mental Health Position Paper on the Report of the Joint Commission on Mental Illness and Health," November 1961, NIMH Records, Miscellaneous Records 1956–1967, Box 1.

49. "Report of [NIMH] Task Force on the Status of State Mental Hospitals in the United States," March 30, 1962, Bertram Brown Papers, NLM, Bethesda, Maryland.

50. "Preliminary Draft Report of NIMH Task Force on Implementation of Recommendations of the Report of the Joint Commission on Mental Illness and Health," January 5, 1962, and "A Proposal for a Comprehensive Mental Health Program to Implement the Findings of the Joint Commission on Mental Illness and Health," April 1962, 10, 12, 34–35, and passim, NIMH Records, Miscellaneous Records, 1956–1967, Box 1.

51. 88-2 Congress, *House Report no. 1488* (March 23, 1962), 34–35.

52. Robert H. Atwell to Director, "Proposals for the President's Mental Health Program—A Report to the Interagency Group Appointed by the President," November 1, 1962, Daniel Patrick Moynihan to Boisfuellet Jones, August 21, 1962, Brown Papers; Foley, *Community Mental Health Legislation*, 40–41.

53. Anthony Celebrezze, W. Willard Wirtz, and J. Gleason to John F. Kennedy, November 30, 1962, White House Central Files, Box 338, Folder HE 1-1, Kennedy Library.

54. 88-1 Congress, *Mental Health. Hearings before a Subcommittee of the Committee on Interstate and Foreign Commerce House of Representatives . . . 1963* (Washington, D.C.: Government Printing Office, 1963), 100–106; Foley, *Community Mental Health Legislation*, 41–44.

55. *Wall Street Journal*, January 15, 1963; Myer Feldman interview, September 21, 1968, vol. 14, 13–15, Kennedy Library. See also the Bertram Brown interview by John Stewart, August 6, 1968, 23, ibid., and Felix interview, August 5, 1964 (OH120), APA Archives.

56. Feldman interview, vol. 14, 24–25; Brown interview, 25, Kennedy Library.

57. *Message from the President of the United States Relative to Mental Illness and Mental Retardation*, 88-1 Congress, House of Representatives Document no. 58 (February 5, 1963).

58. 88-1 Congress, *Mental Illness and Retardation. Hearings before the Subcommittee on Health of the Committee of Labor and Public Welfare United States Senate . . . March 5, 6, and 7, 1963* (Washington, D.C.: Government Printing Office, 1963), 17–19, 41–44, 87–88, and passim.

59. Mike Gorman interview by Daniel Blain, October 7, 1972, Blain Papers, APA Archives; 88-1 Congress, *Mental Health. Hearings . . . House*, 99–106, 341–342.

60. The legislative history of the bill can be followed in Grob, *From Asylum to Community*, 229–233.

61. Public Law 88-164, *U.S. Statutes at Large* 77: (1963) 282–299; Robert H. Felix, "A Model for Comprehensive Mental Health Centers," *American Journal of Public Health* 54 (1964): 1965.

62. Data in this and the preceding paragraph are drawn from a sample of studies produced by the staff of the Biometrics Branch during these years that were relevant to policy. See Morton Kramer, "Long Range Studies of Mental Hospital Patients, an Important Area for Research in Chronic Disease," *Milbank Memorial Fund Quarterly* 31

(1953): 253–264; Kramer, H. Goldstein, R. H. Israel, and N. A. Johnson, *A Historical Study of the Disposition of First Admissions to a State Mental Hospital: Experience of Warren State Hospital during the Period 1916–1950*, U.S. Public Health Service Publication 445 (1955); Kramer, *Facts Needed to Assess Public Health and Social Problems in the Widespread Use of the Tranquilizing Drugs*, Public Health Service Publication 486 (Washington, D.C., 1956); Ben Z. Locke, Kramer, C. E. Timberlake, B. Pasamanick, and D. Smeltzer, "Problems in Interpretation of Patterns of First Admissions to Ohio State Public Mental Hospitals for Patients with Schizophrenic Reactions," APA, *Psychiatric Research Reports* 10 (1958): 172–208; Earl S. Pollack, P. H. Person, Kramer, and Goldstein, *Patterns of Retention, Release, and Death of First Admissions to State Mental Hospitals*, Public Health Service Publication 672 (Washington, D.C., 1959); Kramer, Pollack, and R. W. Redick, "Studies of the Incidence and Prevalence of Hospitalized Mental Disorders in the United States: Current Status and Future Goals," in *Comparative Epidemiology of the Mental Disorders*, ed. Paul H. Hoch and J. Zubin (New York: Grune & Stratton,1961), 56–100; Kramer, *Some Implications of Trends in the Usage of Psychiatric Facilities for Community Mental Health Programs and Related Research*, Public Health Service Publication 1434 (Washington, D.C., 1967); Kramer, "Epidemiology, Biostatistics, and Mental Health Planning," in APA *Psychiatric Research Reports* 22 (1967): 1–68; Kramer, C. Taube, and S. Starr, "Patterns of Use of Psychiatric Facilities by the Aged: Current Status, Trends, and Implications," ibid. 23 (1968): 89–150.

63. For a shrewd and insightful analysis of mental health policy in the 1960s, see Alfred J. Kahn, *Studies in Social Policy and Planning* (New York: Russell Sage Foundation, 1969), 194–242.

64. The regulations can be found in the *Federal Register* 29 (1964): 5951–5956. The writing of the regulations is ably traced in Foley, *Community Mental Health Legislation*, 89–98.

65. S. L. Buker Miller and R. N. Elwell, "The Hospital Improvement Project Grant Program," *Mental Hospitals* 15 (1964): 526–528; Arthur A. Woloshin and H. C. Pomp, "The Gulf between Planning and Implementing Mental Health Programs," *Hospital & Community Psychiatry* 19 (1968): 60–61.

66. Annual Conference of the Surgeon General Public Health Service with State and Territorial Mental Health Authorities, *Proceedings, 1965*, Public Health Service Publication 1355 (Washington, D.C., 1965), 10, 11, 39; 89-1 Congress, *Research Facilities, Mental Health Staffing . . . Hearings before the Committee on Interstate and Foreign Commerce House of Representatives . . . 1965* (Washington, D.C.: Government Printing Office, 1965); Public Law 89-105, *U.S. Statutes at Large* 79 (1965): 427–430; *Federal Register* 31 (March 1, 1966): 3246–3248; Foley, *Community Mental Health Legislation* 103–116.

Chapter 2 — Policy Fragmentation

1. Louis Linn, "The Fourth Psychiatric Revolution," *American Journal of Psychiatry* 124 (1968): 1043–1048; Gerald Caplan, "Community Psychiatry," in *Concepts of Community Psychiatry: A Framework for Training*, ed. Stephen E. Goldston, U.S. Public Health Service, Publication 1319 (1964), 4, 10; Caplan, *Principles of Preventive Psychiatry* (New York: Basic Books, 1964), 16ff.

2. Alan I. Levenson and Bertram S. Brown, "Social Implications of the Community Mental Health Center Concept," paper delivered at the American Psychopathological

Association, February 17, 1967, Brown Papers, National Library of Medicine (NLM), Bethesda, Md.

3. 90-1 Congress, *Mental Health Centers Construction Act Extension: Hearings before the Subcommittee on Public Health and Welfare . . . House . . . 1967* (Washington, D.C.: Government Printing Office, 1967), 13, 18, 82–89; 91-1 Congress, *Community Mental Health Centers Amendments of 1969: Hearings before the Subcommittee on Health . . . Senate . . . 1969* (Washington, D.C.: Government Printing Office, 1969), 17–18, 58, 98–102, 121–134, 140–150; Raymond M. Glasscote et al., *The Community Mental Health Center: An Interim Appraisal* (Washington, D.C.: Joint Information Service, 1969), 5–7; 91-1 Congress, *Community Mental Health Centers Act Extension: Hearings before the Subcommittee on Public Health and Welfare . . . House . . . 1969* (Washington, D.C.: Government Printing Office, 1969), 18–21, 96, 107–140, 148–162, 171–172; Christopher J. Smith, "Geographic Patterns of Funding for Community Mental Health Centers," *Hospital & Community Psychiatry* 35 (1984): 1133–1140.

4. Robert H. Connery et al., *The Politics of Mental Health: Organizing Community Health in Metropolitan Areas* (New York: Columbia University Press, 1968), 479; Raymond M. Glasscote, *The Community Mental Health Center: An Analysis of Existing Models* (Washington, D.C.: Joint Information Service, 1964), 22; August B. Hollingshead and F. C. Redlich, *Social Class and Mental Illness: A Community Study* (New York: Wiley, 1958), 258 and passim; Steven S. Sharfstein, "Will Community Mental Health Survive in the 1980s?," *American Journal of Psychiatry* 135 (1978): 1364–1365.

5. Howard H. Goldman et al., "Community Mental Health Centers and the Treatment of Severe Mental Disorders," *American Journal of Psychiatry* 137 (1980): 83–86.

6. "Report of the Meeting of the Ad Hoc Committee on State Mental Health Program Development October 10–11, 1966," NIMH Records, Subject Files, 1963–1966, Box 12, Record Group 511.2, National Archives (NA), Washington, D.C.; NIMH Statistical Note 67 (1972), and Mental Health Statistical Note no. 160 (1981); Glasscote et al., *The Community Mental Health Center,* 12; W. W. Winslow, "The Changing Role of Psychiatrists in Community Mental Health Centers," *American Journal of Psychiatry* 136 (1979): 24–27; Paul J. Fink and S. P. Weinstein, "Whatever Happened to Psychiatry: The Deprofessionalization of Community Mental Health Centers," *American Journal of Psychiatry* 136 (1979): 406–409; Donald G. Langsley, "The Community Mental Health Center: Does It Treat Patients?," *Hospital & Community Psychiatry* 31 (1980): 815–819; Sharfstein, "Will Community Mental Health Survive in the 1980s?," 1365; James W. Thompson and Rosalyn D. Bass, "Changing Staffing Patterns in Community Mental Health Centers," *Hospital & Community Psychiatry* 35 (1984): 1109; David F. Musto, "Whatever Happened to 'Community Mental Health'?," *Public Interest* 39 (1975): 53–79; Gerald N. Grob, *From Asylum to Community: Mental Health Policy in Modern America* (Princeton: Princeton University Press, 1991), 256–257.

7. David Mechanic and David A. Rochefort, "A Policy of Inclusion for the Mentally Ill," *Health Affairs* 11 (1992): 132–133.

8. William Gronfein, "Incentives and Intentions in Mental Health Policy: A Comparison of the Medicaid and Community Mental Health Programs," *Journal of Health and Social Behavior* 26 (1985): 196; "Whom Are Community Mental Health Centers Serving?," NIMH Statistical Note 67 (1972); Lisa Reichenbach, "The Federal Community

Mental Health Centers Program and the Policy of Deinstitutionalization," chaps. 4–5, study prepared for the NIMH under grant no. MH27738-02.

9. William Gronfein, "Psychotropic Drugs and the Origins of Deinstitutionalization," *Social Problems* 32 (1985): 437–454; J. Sanbourne Bockoven, *Moral Treatment in Community Mental Health* (New York: Springer Publishing Co., 1972), 114–146. A similar situation prevailed in Great Britain, where length of stays of schizophrenic patients declined years before the use of psychotropic drugs. See George W. Brown, M. Bone, B. Dalison, and J. K. Wing, *Schizophrenia and Social Care: A Comparative Follow-Up Study of 339 Schizophrenic Patients* (London: Oxford University Press, 1966), and J. K. Wing and G. W. Brown, *Institutionalism and Schizophrenia: A Comparative Study of Three Mental Hospitals, 1960–1968* (Cambridge: Cambridge University Press, 1970).

10. Medicare (Title XVIII) had two parts. Part A dealt with hospital insurance for the aged; Part B dealt with insurance for physician services. Medicaid (Title XIX) involved grants to states for medical assistance programs for indigent persons.

11. The text of Public Law 89-97 (the 1965 amendments to the Social Security Act that created Medicare and Medicaid) can be found in *U.S. Statutes at Large* 79 (1965): 286–422.

12. NIMH Statistical Note 107 (1974): 146, and Note 146 (1978): 4; Morton Kramer, *Psychiatric Services and the Changing Institutional Scene, 1950–1985*, DHEW Publication no. [ADM] 77-433 (Washington, D.C., 1977), 80; Gronfein, "Incentives and Intentions," 192–206; Howard H. Goldman, N. H. Adams, and C. Taube, "Deinstitutionalization: The Data Demythologized," *Hospital & Community Psychiatry* 34 (1983): 133; Charles A. Kiesler and Amy E. Sibulkin, *Mental Hospitalization: Myths and Facts about a National Crisis* (Newbury Park, Calif.: Sage Publications, 1987), 114–130; General Accounting Office, *Returning the Mentally Disabled to the Community: Government Needs to Do More*, HRD-76–152, (Washington, D.C., 1977), 81; Bruce Vladeck, *Unloving Care: The Nursing Home Tragedy* (New York: Basic Books, 1980).

13. Ronald A. Manderscheid and Marilyn J. Henderson, *Mental Health, United States, 2002*, DHHS Publication no. [SMA] 3938 (Rockville, Md.: Substance Abuse and Mental Health Service Administration, 2004), 245–247; Kiesler and Sibulkin, *Mental Hospitalization*, 60.

14. The publication in 1980 of the third edition of the APA's *Diagnostic and Statistical Manual of Mental Disorders* (more commonly known as *DSM-III*) elevated many common behaviors to the status of distinct pathological entities. This broadened the clientele of the mental health system and thus contributed still further to the tendency to shift services away from individuals with more serious illnesses. See Allan Horwitz, *Creating Mental Illness* (Chicago: University of Chicago Press, 2002).

15. Goldman, Adams, and Taube, "Deinstitutionalization," 130; David Mechanic, *Mental Health and Social Policy: The Emergence of Managed Care*, 4th ed. (Boston: Allyn and Bacon, 1999), 7–14; Carl A. Taube and S. A. Barrett, eds., *Mental Health, United States, 1985*, DHHS Publication no. [ADM] 85-1378 (Washington, D.C., 1985), 54; Manderscheid and Henderson, *Mental Health, United States, 2002*, 331.

16. NIMH Statistical Note 23 (April 1970): 1–4, and Note 154 (September 1980): 12; Goldman, Adams, and Taube, "Deinstitutionalization," 131–132.

17. Goldman, Adams, and Taube, "Deinstitutionalization," 133; Kiesler and Sibulkin, *Mental Hospitalization*, 86, 95; Taube and Barrett, *Mental Health, United States, 1985*, 33, 53.

18. Kiesler and Sibulkin, *Mental Hospitalization*, 86, 95; Taube and Barrett, *Mental Health, United States, 1985*, 53

19. James R. Morrissey, "Family Care for the Mentally Ill: A Neglected Therapeutic Resource," *Social Service Review* 39 (1965): 63–71; Walter E. Barton and W. T. St. John, "Family Care and Outpatient Psychiatry," *American Journal of Psychiatry* 117 (1961): 644–647.

20. Donald M. Carmichael, "Community Aftercare Clinics and Fountain House," in *Rehabilitation of the Mentally Ill: Social and Economic Aspects*, ed. Milton Greenblatt and B. Simon (Washington, D.C.: American Association for the Advancement of Science, 1959), 157–178.

21. Ibid., 169–172; Raymond M. Glasscote et al., *Rehabilitating the Mentally Ill in the Community: A Study of Psychosocial Rehabilitation Centers* (Washington, D.C.: Joint Information Service, 1971), 8, 19–20, 41–63, 175–177; Glasscote et al., *Halfway Houses for the Mentally Ill: A Study of Programs and Problems* (Washington, D.C.: Joint Information Service, 1971), 10–24; Harold L. Raush and C. L. Raush, *The Halfway House Movement: A Search for Sanity* (New York: Appleton Century Crofts, 1968); Naomi D. Rothwell and J. M. Doniger, *The Psychiatric Halfway House: A Case Study* (Springfield, Ill.: Charles C. Thomas, 1966).

22. Thomas. S. Szasz, *The Myth of Mental Illness: Foundations of a Theory of Personal Conduct* (New York: Hoeber-Harper, 1961), and *Law, Liberty, and Psychiatry: An Inquiry into the Social Uses of Mental Health Practices* (New York: Macmillan, 1963); R. D. Laing, *Sanity, Madness, and the Family* (London: Tavistock, 1964), and *The Politics of Experience and the Bird of Paradise* (New York: Pantheon Books, 1967); Erving Goffman, *Asylums: Essays on the Social Situation of Mental Patients and Other Inmates* (Garden City, N.Y.: Anchor Books, 1961); Thomas J. Scheff, *Being Mentally Ill: A Sociological Theory* (Chicago: Aldine Publishing Co., 1966), and "Schizophrenia as Ideology," *Schizophrenia Bulletin*, 2 (Fall 1970): 15–19.

23. Roy R. Grinker, Sr., "Emerging Concepts of Mental Illness and Models of Treatment: The Medical Point of View," George W. Albee, "Emerging Concepts of Mental Illness and Models of Treatment: The Psychological Point of View," and "Letters to the Editor," *American Journal of Psychiatry* 125 (1969): 870–876, 1744–1746.

24. Morton Birnbaum, "The Right to Treatment," *American Bar Association Journal* 46 (1960): 499–505; 87-1 Congress, *Constitutional Rights of the Mentally Ill: Hearings before the Subcommittee on Constitutional Rights of the Committee on the Judiciary . . . Senate . . . 1961* (Washington, D.C.: Government Printing Office, 1961), 2, 273–305.

25. Bruce Ennis, *Prisoners of Psychiatry: Mental Patients, Psychiatrists, and the Law* (New York: Harcourt Brace Jovanovich, 1972), vii–viii. See also Ennis and L. Siegel, *The Rights of Mental Patients: The Basic ACLU Guide to a Mental Patient's Rights* (New York: Richard W. Baron, 1973).

26. See Alexander D. Brooks, *Law, Psychiatry and the Mental Health System* (Boston: Little, Brown, 1974) and the *1980 Supplement* (Boston: Little, Brown, 1980) to this volume.

27. Paul S. Appelbaum, *Almost a Revolution: Mental Health Law and the Limits of Change* (New York: Oxford University Press, 1994), 142–146, 211–212; David Mechanic, "Judicial Action and Social Change," in *The Right to Treatment for Mental Patients*, ed. Stuart Golann and William J. Fremouw (New York: Irvington Publishers, 1976), 47–72. See also Rael Jean and V. C. Armat, *Madness in the Streets: How*

Psychiatry and the Law Abandoned the Mentally Ill (New York: Free Press, 1990), and Alan A. Stone's *Mental Health and the Law: A System in Transition* (New York: Jason Aronson, 1976), "Overview: The Right to Treatment—Comments on the Law and Its Impact," *American Journal of Psychiatry* 132 (1975): 1125–1134, and *Law, Psychiatry, and Morality* (Washington, D.C.: American Psychiatric Press, 1984).

28. U.S. Bureau of the Census, *Historical Statistics of the United States: Colonial Times to 1970*, 2 vols. (Washington, D.C.: Government Printing Office, 1975), 1:49; Kramer, *Psychiatric Services and the Changing Institutional Scene*, 46; Leona L. Bachrach, "Young Adult Chronic Patients: An Analytical Review of the Literature," *Hospital & Community Psychiatry* 33 (1982): 189–197.

29. Bert Pepper, H. Ryglewicz, and M. C. Kirschner, "The Uninstitutionalized Generation: A New Breed of Psychiatric Patient," in *The Young Adult Chronic Patient*, ed. Pepper and Ryglewicz (San Francisco: Jossey-Bass, 1982), 5. See also Leona L. Bachrach, "The Homeless Mentally Ill and Mental Health Services: An Analytical Review of the Literature," in *The Homeless Mentally Ill: A Task Force Report of the American Psychiatric Association*, ed. H. Richard Lamb (Washington, D.C.: American Psychiatric Association, 1984), 11–53.

30. Leona L. Bachrach, "The Concept of Young Adult Chronic Psychiatric Patients: Questions from a Research Perspective," *Hospital & Community Psychiatry* 35 (1984): 574; H. Richard Lamb, "Deinstitutionalization and the Homeless Mentally Ill," in Lamb, *The Homeless Mentally Ill*, 65.

31. Stuart R. Schwartz and S. M. Goldfinger, "The New Chronic Patient: Clinical Characteristics of an Emerging Subgroup," *Hospital & Community Psychiatry* 32 (1981): 473. See especially the essays in *Barriers to Treating the Chronic Mentally Ill*, ed. Arthur T. Meyerson (San Francisco: Jossey-Bass, 1987).

32. 90-2 Congress, *Departments of Labor, and Health, Education, and Welfare Appropriations for Fiscal Year 1969: Hearings before the Subcommittee of the Committee on Appropriations United States Senate* (Washington, D.C.: Government Printing Office, 1968), 612–613; 91-1 Congress, *Departments of Labor, and Health, Education, and Welfare Appropriations for 1970: Hearings before the Subcommittee of the Committee on Appropriations House of Representatives* (Washington, D.C.: Government Printing Office, 1969), part 2, 10.

33. Langsley, "The Community Mental Health Center: Does It Treat Patients?," 815–819; Rosalyn D. Bass, *CMHC Staffing: Who Minds the Store?*, DHEW Publ. [ADM] 78-686 (Washington, D.C., 1978).

34. See Stephan P. Strickland, *Politics, Science, and Dread Disease: A Short History of United States Medical Research Policy* (Cambridge: Harvard University Press, 1972), and Grob, *From Asylum to Community*. A good description of the biomedical lobby can be found in Elizabeth B. Drew, "The Health Syndicate: Washington's Noble Conspirators," *Atlantic Monthly* 220 (December 1967): 75–82.

35. The fight between the administration and Congress can be followed in a number of committee hearings. See especially 92-2 Congress, *Extend Community Mental Health Centers Act: Hearing before the Subcommittee on Public Health and Environment of the Committee on Interstate and Foreign Commerce House of Representatives . . . 1972* (Washington, D.C.: Government Printing Office, 1972); 93-1 Congress, *Public Health Service Act Extension, 1973: Hearing before the Committee on Labor and Welfare United States Senate . . . 1973* (Washington, D.C.: Government Printing Office, 1973); and 93-1 Congress, *Departments of Labor, and Health, Education and*

Welfare and Related Agencies Appropriations for Fiscal Year 1974: Hearings before a Subcommittee of the Committee on Appropriations United States Senate (Washington, D.C.: Government Printing Office, 1973) (the Weinberger statement appeared in part 1, 91–92). For analyses of the policy debates of the early 1970s, see Henry A. Foley, *Community Mental Health Legislation: The Formative Process* (Lexington, Mass.: Lexington Books, 1975); Walter E. Barton and Charlotte J. Sanborn, eds., *An Assessment of the Community Mental Health Movement* (Lexington, Mass.: Lexington Books, 1977); Henry A. Foley and Steven S. Sharfstein, *Madness and Government: Who Cares for the Mentally Ill?* (Washington, D.C.: American Psychiatric Press, 1983); E. Fuller Torrey, *Nowhere to Go: The Tragic Odyssey of the Homeless Mentally Ill* (New York: Harper & Row, 1988); and Reichenbach, "The Federal Community Mental Health Centers Program and the Policy of Deinstitutionalization."

36. General Accounting Office, "Need for More Effective Management of Community Mental Health Centers Program," August 27, 1974 (Government Document B-164031[5]), iii. See also this agency's earlier report, "Community Mental Health Centers Program—Improvements Needed in Management," July 8, 1971 (B-164031[2]).

37. Public Law 94-63, *U.S. Statutes at Large* 89 (July 29, 1975): 304–369, Public Law 95-83, ibid. 91 (August 1, 1977): 383–399, and Public Law 95-622, ibid. 92 (November 9, 1978): 3412–3442.

38. General Accounting Office, *Returning the Mentally Disabled to the Community: Government Needs to Do More*, January 7, 1977 (HRD-76-152), viii, 19–25, 28, 44, 72.

39. Ibid., 81, 119, 128, 137, 154.

40. Ibid., 172–182.

41. Ibid., 184–191.

42. Ibid., 184, 192–203.

Chapter 3 — A Presidential Initiative

1. See David Flitner, Jr., *The Politics of Presidential Commissions* (Dobbs Ferry, N.Y.: Transnational Publishers, 1986), and Amy B. Zegart, "Blue Ribbons, Black Boxes: Toward a Better Understanding of Presidential Commissions," *Presidential Studies Quarterly* 34 (June 2004): 366–391.

2. Joyce Gallagher interview with Rosalynn Carter, December 21, 1974, Jimmy Carter Presidential Library, Atlanta, Georgia (JCPL), 10–15; Rosalynn Carter, *First Lady from Plains* (Boston: Houghton Mifflin Co., 1984), 95–97.

3. See Kandy Stroud, "Rosalynn's Agenda in the White House," *New York Times Magazine*, March 20, 1977, 19–20, 58–59; *New York Times*, March 10, 1977, 18, June 5, 1944, E4, February 14, 1978, 20, May 30, 1978, B1; B. Drummond Ayres, Jr., "The Importance of Being Rosalynn," *New York Times Magazine*, June 3, 1979, 39–41, 43–44, 46, 48, 50, 56. See also Carter, *First Lady*.

4. Gerald N. Grob interview with Thomas E. Bryant (TEB), April 11, 2003.

5. Ibid; Gerald N. Grob interview with Beatrix Hamburg, November 25, 2003.

6. White House Press Secretary Release, "Executive Order. President's Commission on Mental Health," February 17, 1977, Box 25, Presidential Commission on Mental Health Papers, Record Group 25, JCPL (hereafter PCMH Papers).

7. TEB interview; *Psychiatric News* 12 (March 18, 1977): 14.

8. Gerald N. Grob interview with Paul Danaceau, December 12, 2003.

9. TEB interview; Office of the First Lady's Press Secretary, PCMH, Fact Sheet, April 19, 1977, Box 25, PCMH Papers; *Psychiatric News* 12 (May 6, 1977): 1, 12.

10. See, for example, TEB to Senator John Melcher, April 28, 1977; TEB to Representative Bill Alexander, October 28, 1977, Box 22, PCMH Papers.

11. TEB interview.

12. Detailed résumés of each commissioner can be found in Boxes 20 and 21, PCMH Papers.

13. *Psychiatric News* 12 (May 6, 1977), 13.

14. "Notes on Briefing of Commissioners-Designate of President's Commission on Mental Health, March 29, 1977," 1–12, Box 1, PCMH Papers.

15. TEB interview; TEB to Margaret McKenna, April 5, Joseph A. Califano, Jr., to TEB, April 28, TEB to James Dickson, April 29, 1977, Box 22, PCMH Papers.

16. TEB Memo to Margaret McKenna, April 5, TEB to James B. Rielly, April 26, TEB Memo to Ben Heineman, Jr., May 3, 1977, Box 22, TEB to Hugh A. Carter, Jr., February 22, 1978, Box 24, PCMH Papers; Danaceau interview; TEB interview.

17. TEB interview.

18. Gerald N. Grob interview with Gary L. Tischler, November 3, 2003.

19. "President's Commission on Mental Health—Task Panels Announced," June 16, 1977, Box 25; Information Bulletin, July 20, 1977, Box 25; Richard A. Millstein to Paul R. Friedman, November 15, 1977, Box 23, PCMH Papers; *Psychiatric News* 12 (July 15, 1977): 1, 6. A list of the members of the task panels as well as their reports can be found in volumes 2, 3, and 4 of the *Report to the President from the President's Commission on Mental Health,* 4 vols. (Washington, D.C.: Government Printing Office, 1978).

20. Vic Pfeiffer to TEB, June 9, 1977, Box 22; "Congressional Responses to letter sent by PCMH," n.d., Box 22, PCMH Papers.

21. TEB to Priscilla Allen, April 12, 1977, Box 22, PCMH Papers. Identical letters were sent to all commissioners.

22. Priscilla Allen, "A Consumer's View of California's Mental Health Care system," *Psychiatric Quarterly* 48, no. 1 (1974): 2–4. Allen was critical of the generalization that hospital care was always "bad" and community care "good." Many discharged patients led bleak and isolated lives in the community. Indeed, community care and treatment, she insisted, "may actually mean *less real participation* than a person would enjoy 'confined' within an out-of-the-community state hospital."

23. The summary of the discussions in this and the preceding paragraph is drawn from "Meeting of the President's Commission on Mental Health . . . April 19, 1977," 19–21, 25–29, 48–53, 60–64, 74–83, 89–99, Box 1, PCMH Papers.

24. "Gathering Information and Data: Staff and Panel Work Plans," April 19, 1977, Box 1; "Dr. Bryant's Remarks at the June 16, 1977 Press Conference," Box 25, PCMH Papers.

25. Verbatim transcripts are found in "President's Commission on Mental Health. Philadelphia, Pennsylvania, May 24, 1977," Box 10; "Public Hearing before the President's Commission on Mental Health [Nashville, May 25, 1977]," Box 12; "A Public Hearing before the President's Commission on Mental Health . . . Tucson, Arizona . . . June 20, 1977," Box 14; "The President's Commission on Mental Health. Public Hearing, San Francisco, California . . . June 21, 1977," Box 17, PCMH Papers.

26. Soffer's testimony can be found in "President's Commission on Mental Health. Philadelphia . . . May 24, 1977," 57–64. A summary can be found in *Psychiatric News* 12 (July 1, 1977): 8, 15.

27. "Public Hearing . . . [Nashville]," 9–14; "A Public Hearing . . . Tucson," 20–26, 29–34, 54–55, 60–61; "The President's Commission . . . San Francisco," 18–21; *Psychiatric News* 12 (July 1, 1977): 9, 15.

28. These generalizations are based on a reading of the verbatim transcripts of the four public hearings cited above. Lanterman's testimony can be found in "The President's Commission . . . San Francisco," 239–246.

29. *New York Times,* March 10, 18, May 25, 1977, A16, June 5, 1977, E4, August 26, 1977, A4, November 6, 1977, 1, 21; *Los Angeles Times,* April 21, 1977, part IV, 1, 6; *Washington Post,* August 27, 1977, 12; Rosalynn Carter, "Removing the Mental-Illness Stigma," *New York Times,* November 18, 1977, A31; Rosalynn Carter, "Toward a More Caring Society," *MH* 61 (Summer-Fall 1977): 1–5; Joel Greenberg, "Not Just for Show," *Science News* 111 (June 18, 1977): 396–397; Ayres, "The Importance of Being Rosalynn," 39–41, 43–44, 46, 48, 50, 56.

30. "Public Meeting, Commissioner's Meeting . . . June 22, 1977," passim, and "Summary," 1–3, Box 1; Virginia Dayton to TEB, May 27, 1977, Rev. Franklin E. Vilas, Jr., to TEB, May 31, 1977, Charles V. Willie Memos to PCMH, June ?, 24, 1977, Box 21, John Conger to TEB, July 15, 1977, Box 20, PCMH Papers; *Psychiatric News* 12 (August 5, 1977): 1, 9–11.

31. "Public Meeting, Commissioner's Meeting . . . June 22, 1977," 9–10, 26–28, 52–55.

32. See Steven S. Sharfstein, Judith E. Clark Turner, and Harry W. Clark, "Financing Issues in the Delivery of Services to the Chronically Mentally Ill and Disabled," in *The Chronic Mental Patient: Problems, Solutions, and Recommendations for a Public Policy Prepared by the Ad Hoc Committee on the Chronic Mental Patient,* ed. John A. Talbott (Washington, D.C.: American Psychiatric Association, 1978), 137–150; Gerald N. Grob interview with Steven S. Sharfstein, October 24, 2003.

33. Talbott, *The Chronic Mental Patient,* xiv–xv, 211–220.

34. "Meeting of the President's Commission on Mental Health July 11–12, 1977 . . . Summary," Box 1; "Meeting of the President's Commission on Mental Health . . . August 2–3, 1977 . . . Summary," Box 2, PCMH Papers.

35. "Transcript of Proceedings . . . Meeting on Prevention . . . 3 August 1977," 5–10, 47, 50–51, Box 3; "Meeting of the President's Commission on Mental Health . . . August 2–3, 1977 . . . Summary," 1–3, Box 2, PCMH Papers.

36. "Transcript of Proceedings . . . Meeting on Mental Health Manpower . . . 2 August 1977," 23–24, Box 3, PCMH Papers. All of the transcripts of the individual sessions can be found in Box 3, PCMH Papers.

37. *Psychiatric News* 12 (August 19, 1977): 1, 10–11.

38. TEB to Peter Bourne, September 8, 1977, Box 23, PCMH Papers.

39. Beverly Long to Beatrix Hamburg, July 16, 1977, Long to TEB, August 17, 1977, LaDonna Harris to TEB, August 26, 1977, Thomas L. Conlan to PCMH, July 1, 1977, Conlon Notes telephoned to TEB, August 9, 1977, Box 21, PCMH Papers.

40. TEB to Priscilla Allen, September 15, 1977 (similar letters sent to all commissioners), Box 23; "Washington Press Club—September 15, 1977, Mrs. Carter's Remarks," Box 25, PCMH Papers.

41. "Preliminary Report to the President from the President's Commission on Mental Health September 1, 1977," 1–7, Box 2, PCMH Papers.

42. Ibid., 8–10.

43. Ibid., 9–22.

44. *Psychiatric News* 12 (September 16, 1977): 1.

45. *Mental Health Reports* 1 (September 12, 1977):1–2, Box 25; "Transcript of Proceedings President's Commission on Mental Health . . . 14 October 1977," 110–119, Box 4, PCMH Papers; E. Fuller Torrey, "Carter's Little Pills," *Psychology Today* 11 (December 1977): 10, 12; TEB to Editor, *Psychology Today,* November 30, 1977, Box 24, PCMH Papers.

46. "Meeting of the President's Commission on Mental Health . . . October 14–15, 1977 . . . Summary," 1–6, Box 4, PCMH Papers.

47. "Meeting of the President's Commission on Mental Health December 9–10, 1977 . . . Summary," 1–2, Box 4; "Transcript of Proceedings President's Commission on Mental Health . . . December 9, 1977," 4–52, Box 5, PCMH Papers.

48. Memo from Richard H. Millstein to George Albee, December 12, 1977, Box 24, PCMH Papers.

49. "Transcript of Proceedings of the President's Commission on Mental Health, December 9, 1977," 53–60, 103–111, 133–138; "Meeting of the President's Commission on Mental Health December 9–10, 1977 . . . Summary," 2–11; "Transcript of Proceedings President's Commission on Mental Health . . . December 10, 1977," 177, 183, 199–200, 202–18, 226–227, Box 5, PCMH Papers.

50. "Transcript of Proceedings President's Commission on Mental Health . . . January 16, 1978," 5–20, "Transcript of Proceedings President's Commission on Mental Health . . . January 17, 1978; "Meeting of the President's Commission on Mental Health January 16–17, 1978 . . . Summary," Box 6, PCMH Papers.

51. The task panel reports appeared in vols. 2, 3, and 4 of the *Report to the President from the President's Commission on Mental Health.* They were as follows: Mental Health—Nature and Scope of the Problems; Community Support Systems; Planning and Review; Organization and Structure; Community Mental Health Centers Assessment; Access and Barriers to Care; Deinstitutionalization, Rehabilitation and Long-Term Care; Alternative Services—A Special Study; Mental Health Personnel; Cost and Financing; Mental Health of American Families General Issues and Adult Years; Infants, Children, Adolescents; Learning Failure and Unused Learning Potential; Special Populations; Mental Health of Minorities, Women, Physically Handicapped; Mental Health of the Elderly; Rural Mental Health; Migrant and Seasonal Farmworkers; Mental Health Problems of Vietnam Era Veterans—A Study; Legal and Ethical Issues; Research; Prevention; Public Attitudes and Use of Media for Promotion of Mental Health; Arts in Therapy and Environment; State Mental Health Issues. In addition, there were three liaison task panel reports: Mental Retardation; Alcohol-Related Problems; Psychoactive Drug Use/Misuse.

52. "Report of the Task Panel on the Nature and Scope of the Problems," in *Report to the President,* 2:1–138.

53. *Report to the President,* 3:730–1358.

54. Ibid., 4:1359–1516.

55. Ibid., 2:139–135, 275–311, 340–375, 497–544.

56. Ibid., 2:312–339.

57. Ibid., 2:236–274, 376–496, 3:545–729, 4:1517–1924, 1991–2140.

Chapter 4 — From Advocacy to Legislation

1. Thomas L. Conlan to Thomas E. Bryant (TEB), March 9, 1978, Conlan to PCMH Commissioners, n.d. ("Suggestions for consideration in setting the tone . . . of our Report"), Charles V. Willie to TEB, February 2, 1978, Beverly B. Long to Rosalynn Carter

and TEB, February 11, 1978, Box 21; Allan Beigel to TEB, December 15, 1977, Priscilla Allen to Mildred Starin, December 2, 1977, Allen to Gary Tischler, February 20, 1978, Box 20; Martha Mitchell to TEB, March 20, 1978, Box 21, Presidential Commission on Mental Health Papers, Record Group 25, Jimmy Carter Presidential Library, Atlanta, Georgia (hereafter PCMH Papers); Gerald N. Grob interview with Paul Danaceau, December 12, 2003; Gerald N. Grob interview with TEB, April 11, 2003.

2. Memo, TEB to all commissioners, February 7, 1978, Box 9, PCMH Papers.

3. "Transcript of Proceedings President's Commission on Mental Health . . . February 17, 18. 1978," 3–18, Box 7, PCMH Papers.

4. Danaceau interview. The commission's deliberations and debates over the wording of the final report can be followed in "Transcript of Proceeding President's Commission on Mental Health . . . February 17, 18, 1978," Box 7, and "Transcript of Proceedings President's Commission on Mental Health," March 6, 7, 8, 1978, Box 8, PCMH Papers.

5. *Report to the President from the President's Commission on Mental Health,* 4 vols. (Washington, D.C.: Government Printing Office, 1978), 1:3–4.

6. Ibid., 4–9.

7. Ibid., 12–15.

8. Ibid., 16–28, 64–65.

9. Ibid., 29–34.

10. Ibid., 35–41.

11. Ibid., 42–45.

12. Ibid., 46–50, 55–57.

13. Ibid., 51–64.

14. The PCMH, although it had liaison task panels on alcoholism, the misuse of psychoactive drugs, and mental retardation, felt that each of these problems required separate action.

15. Henry A. Foley and Steven S. Sharfstein, *Madness and Government: Who Cares for the Mentally Ill?* (Washington, D.C.: American Psychiatric Press, 1983), 112–116 (both authors were involved in the policymaking process during this period, and their book is actually a primary source document); Gerald N. Grob interview with Steven S. Sharfstein, October 24, 2003; Gerald N. Grob interview with Gary L. Tischler, November 3, 2003.

16. Office of the White House Secretary, "Remarks of the President upon Receiving Final Report of the President's Commission on Mental Health," Box 25, PCMH Papers.

17. *New York Times,* April 22, 1977, A17, August 4, 1977, 22, September 16, 1977, A16; *Washington Post,* September 16, 1977, A4; "Mental Illness Rx: Research, Insurance," *Science News* 112 (September 24, 1977): 198–199; Constance Holden, "Mental Health," *Science* 198 (October 7, 1977): 37.

18. Ron McMillen, "In the Public Eye: Psychiatry in the Mass Media," *Psychiatric News,* 12 (November 18, 1977): 32.

19. Mildred K. Lehman to Earl Ubell, September 20, 1977, TEB to Richard Walk, September 23, 1977, Box 23, PCMH Papers.

20. *Washington Post,* April 28, 1978, A1, 22; *Wall Street Journal,* April 28, 1978, 1; *Science News* 113 (May 6, 1978): 293; Barbara Armstrong, "The Report of the President's Commission on Mental Health: A Summary of Recommendations," *Hospital & Community Psychiatry* 29 (1978): 468–474; Frank Riessman, "The President's Commission on Mental Health: The Self-Help Prospect," *Social Policy* 9 (May–June

1978): 28–31; Alvin L. Schorr, "Mental Health Misfire," *New York Times,* July 24, 1978, A17; idem, "The President's Commission on Mental Health as a Symptom," *American Journal of Orthopsychiatry* 49 (1979): 388–391.

21. *Psychiatric News* 13 (1978): 1, 8–9, 35; *Hospital & Community Psychiatry* 29 (1978): 348–349.

22. Foley and Sharfstein, *Madness and Government,* 118.

23. Leonard I. Stein and Mary Ann Test, "Alternative to Mental Hospital Treatment. I. Conceptual Model, Treatment Program, and Clinical Evaluation," *Archives of General Psychiatry* 37 (1980): 392–397; Burton A. Weisbrod, Test, and Stein, "Alternative to Mental Hospital Treatment. II. Economic Benefit-Cost Analysis," ibid., 400–405; Test and Stein, "Alternative to Mental Hospital Treatment. III. Social Cost," ibid., 409–412; Kenneth S. Thompson, E. E. H. Griffith, and P. J. Leaf, "A Historical Review of the Madison Model of Community Care," and Mark Olfson, "Assertive Community Treatment: An Evaluation of the Experimental Evidence," *Hospital & Community Psychiatry* 41 (1990): 625–641.

24. Judith Clark Turner and William J. TenHoor, "The NIMH Community Support Program: Pilot Approach to a Needed Social Reform," *Schizophrenia Bulletin* 4 (1978): 319–345. See also National Institute of Mental Health Community Support Program, *Report of the Learning Community Conferences June 30, 1979,* mimeographed report prepared by J. A. Reyes Associates, Inc., Washington, D.C.

25. Foley and Sharfstein, *Madness and Government,* 118–119; *Report of the HEW Task Force of the Report to the President from the President's Commission on Mental Health December 15, 1978,* HEW Publication no. (ADM)79-848 (1979), app. 2.

26. *Report of the HEW Task Force,* Executive Summary, 3–11, app. 4, 1–33.

27. *Report to the President from the President's Commission on Mental Health,* 1:22–23; *Report of the HEW Task Force,* Executive Summary, Correction Sheet (preceding p. ES-1), B-3–4.

28. *Psychiatric News* 13 (November 3, 1978): 3, 9.

29. TEB, Public Committee on Mental Health (Washington, D.C.: n.p., 1979), cited in Foley and Sharfstein, *Madness and Government,* 119.

30. *Mental Health Systems. Message from the President of the United States,* 96-1 Congress, House Document no. 96-125 (Washington, D.C.: Government Printing Office, 1979), 1–4.

31. Ibid., 5–56.

32. Stephen M. Rose, "Deciphering Deinstitutionalization: Complexities in Policy and Program Analysis," *Milbank Memorial Fund Quarterly* 57 (1979): 440. See also Ernest M. Gruenberg and Janet Archer, "Abandonment of Responsibility for the Seriously Mentally Ill," *ibid.,* 485–506, and Edward M. Kennedy, "Community Mental Health Care: New Services from Old Systems," ibid., 480–484.

33. For examples, see the following: Charles Windle and Diana Scully, "Community Mental Health Centers and the Decreasing Use of State Mental Hospitals," *Community Mental Health Journal* 12 (1976): 229–243; Howard M. Kaplan and Ronald H. Bohr, "Changes in the Mental Health Field?," *ibid.,* 244–251; NIMH, *Community Mental Health Centers: The Federal Involvement,* HEW Publication no. [ADM] 78-677 (1978); Steven S. Sharfstein, "Will Community Mental Health Survive in the 1980s?," *American Journal of Psychiatry,* 135 (1978): 1363–1365; idem, "Community Mental Health Centers: Returning to Basics," ibid. 136 (1979): 1077–1079; Allan Beigel, Steven Sharfstein, and John C. Wolfe, "Toward Increased Psychiatric

Presence in Community Mental Health Centers," *Hospital & Community Psychiatry* 30 (1979): 763–767.

34. 96-1 Congress, *Reappraisal of Mental Health Policy, 1979: Hearing before the Subcommittee on Health and Scientific Research of the Committee on Labor and Human Resources United States Senate . . . February 7, 1979* (Washington, D.C.: Government Printing Office, 1979), 5–8, 11–19; *Washington Post,* February 8, 1979, A2.

35. 96-1 Congress, *Reappraisal of Mental Health Policy, 1979: Hearing before the Subcommittee on Health and Scientific Research of the Committee on Labor and Human Resources United States Senate,* 1–3.

36. Kennedy, "Community Mental Health Care," 480–484.

37. See Burton Hersh, *The Shadow President: Ted Kennedy in Opposition* (South Royalton, Vt: Steerforth Press, 1997), 32–53.

38. 96-1 Congress, *Mental Health Systems Act, 1979: Hearings before the Subcommittee on Health and Scientific Research of the Committee in Labor and Human Resources United States Senate . . . 1979* (Washington, D.C.: Government Printing Office, 1980), 54–69.

39. This summary was the one subsequently presented by the Senate Committee on Labor and Human Resources when it introduced a revised version of the bill in May, 1980. 96-2 Congress, *Senate Report no. 96-712* (May 15, 1980), 40.

40. 96-1 Congress, *Mental Health Systems Act, 1979: Hearings before the Subcommittee on Health and Scientific Research of the Committee on Labor and Human Resources United States Senate,* 70–72, 116–120, 138, 152–156, 190–203, 227–253, 260–293.

41. Ibid., 293–330, 458–557; *Psychiatric News,* 14 (July 6, 1979): 1, 6–7, 10.

42. 96-1 Congress, *Mental Health Systems Act: Hearings before the Subcommittee on Health and the Environment of the Committee on Interstate and Foreign Commerce House of Representatives . . . 1979* (Washington, D.C.: Government Printing Office, 1979), 64–83.

43. Ibid., 86–248, 328–354.

44. Foley and Sharfstein, *Madness and Government,* 123–124.

45. Ibid., 124.

46. Ibid., 125–126; 96-2 Congress, *Senate Report no. 96-712,* 3–5, 40.

47. Foley and Sharfstein, *Madness and Government,* 126–127.

48. 96-1 Congress, *Community Support for Mental Patients. Hearing Before the Subcommittee on Health and the Environment of the Committee in Interstate and Foreign Commerce House of Representatives . . . 1979* (Washington, D.C.: Government Printing Office, 1979), 62–76.

49. Ibid., 92–115.

50. 96-2 Congress, *Community Mental Health Centers Program Oversight. Hearing before the Subcommittee on Health and the Environment of the Committee on Interstate and Foreign Commerce House of Representatives . . . 1980* (Washington, D.C.: Government Printing Office, 1980), 3–28.

51. 96-2 Congress, *House Report no. 96–977* (May 15, 1980), 1–47.

52. 96-2 Congress, *Congressional Record,* 126, part 15, 19472–19524; *Psychiatric News* 15 (February 1, 1980): 1, 4.

53. 96-2 Congress, *Congressional Record,* 126, part 17, 22692–22734.

54. Foley and Sharfstein, *Madness and Government,* 128–129. A third point of dispute (concerning the administration rather than the Congress) was the inclusion in the House bill of a provision that provided additional physician bonuses in the Public

Health Service comparable to those included in a recently enacted military pay bill. The Office of Management and Budget was opposed, but the amendment was included in the final bill.

55. 96-2 Congress, *House Report no. 96-1367* (September 22, 1980), 62–63.
56. 96-2 Congress, *Congressional Record,* 126, part 20, 26511–26528, part 21, 28382–28387, 28412; 96-2 Congress, *Senate Report no. 96-980* (September 23, 1980); *New York Times,* October 8, 1980, B6.
57. For an important analysis of the Mental Health Systems Act by Sharfstein (who was involved in the writing of the legislation), see Foley and Sharfstein, *Madness and Government,* 130–134.
58. Public Law 96-398, *U.S. Statutes at Large* 94 (1980): 1564–1613; *Psychiatric News* 15 (November 7, 1980): 1, 18–19.
59. Foley and Sharfstein, *Madness and Government,* 137–140.
60. Public Law 97-35, *U.S. Statutes at Large* 95 (1981): 535–598; *Psychiatric News* 16 (March 20, 1981): 1, 11 (April 3, 1981): 1, 28–29 (August 21, 1981): 1, 23; Bruce Bower, "What Reagan Learned in California," ibid., 16 (November 6, 1981): 3.
61. David Mechanic, *Mental Health and Social Policy: The Emergence of Managed Care,* 4th ed. (Boston: Allyn and Bacon, 1999), 98–99.
62. Department of Health and Human Services Steering Committee on the Chronically Mentally Ill, *Toward a National Plan for the Chronically Mentally Ill* (Washington, D.C.: U. S. Public Health Service, 1980), ES1–ES17; Chris Koyanagi and Howard H. Goldman, "The Quiet Success of the National Plan for the Chronically Mentally Ill," *Hospital & Community Psychiatry* 42 (1991): 899–905; Koyanagi and Goldman, *Inching Forward: A Report on Progress Made in Federal Mental Health Policy in the 1980's* (Alexandria, Va.: National Mental Health Association, 1991), 7–53.
63. Daniel X. Freedman, "The President's Commission: Realistic Remedies for Neglect," *Archives of General Psychiatry* 35 (June 1978): 675–676; Darrel A. Regier, Irving D. Goldberg, and Carl A. Taube, "The De Facto U.S. Mental Health Services System," ibid., 685–693; Lee N. Robins, "Psychiatric Epidemiology," ibid., 697–702.
64. American Psychiatric Association, *Diagnostic and Statistical Manual of Mental Disorders,* 3rd ed. (Washington, D.C.: American Psychiatric Association, 1980).

Chapter 5 — From Legislative Repeal to Sequential Reform

1. William Greider, "The Education of David Stockman," *Atlantic* 248 (December 1981): 27–54.
2. Howard H. Goldman, "The Obligation to the Least Well-Off in Mental Health Services," *Psychiatric Services* 50 (1999): 659–663.
3. Department of Health and Human Services Steering Committee on the Chronically Mentally Ill, *Toward a National Plan for the Chronically Mentally Ill* (Washington, D.C.: U.S. Public Health Service, 1980); Chris Koyanagi and Howard H. Goldman, "The Quiet Success of the National Plan for the Chronically Mentally Ill," *Hospital & Community Psychiatry* 42 (1991): 899–905; Chris Koyanagi and Howard Goldman, *Inching Forward: A Report on Progress Made in Federal Mental Health Policy in the 1980's* (Alexandria, Va.: National Mental Health Association, 1991), 7–53.
4. The construct and term "sequentialism" is introduced in Kevin D. Hennessy and Howard H. Goldman, "Full Parity: Steps Toward Treatment Equity for Mental and Addictive Disorders," *Health Affairs* 20 (2001): 58–67, and in Howard H. Goldman, "Vooruitstrevend GGZ-Beleid in Conservatieve Tijden," *Maanblad Geestelijke*

Volksgezondheit 59 (2004): 417–427 ["Making Progress in Mental Health Policy in Conservative Times," paper written based on the Arie Querido lecture in Amsterdam, Netherlands, October 2003, and translated from English]. An abbreviated English version of this paper will appear as "Progress in Mental Health Policy in Conservative Times: One Step at a Time," in *Schizophrenia Bulletin* in 2006.

5. Howard H. Goldman and Gerald N. Grob, "Defining Mental Illness in Mental Health Policy," *Health Affairs* 25 (2006): 737–749.

6. Judith Clark Turner and William J. TenHoor, "The NIMH Community Support Program: Pilot Approach to a Needed Social Reform," *Schizophrenia Bulletin* 4 (1978): 319–345.

7. Joseph P. Morrissey and Howard H. Goldman, "Cycles of Reform in the Care of the Chronically Mentally Ill," *Hospital & Community Psychiatry* 35 (1984): 785–793; Howard H. Goldman and Joseph P. Morrissey, "The Alchemy of Mental Health Policy: Homelessness and the Fourth Cycle of Reform," *American Journal of Public Health* 75 (1985): 727–731.

8. General Accounting Office, *Returning the Mentally Disabled to the Community: Government Needs to Do More*, January 7, 1977 (HRD-76-152); David F. Musto, "Whatever Happened to 'Community Mental Health'?," *Public Interest*, 39 (1975): 53–79; Donald G. Langsley, "The Community Mental Health Center: Does It Treat Patients?," *Hospital & Community Psychiatry* 31 (1980): 815–819; Howard H. Goldman et al., "Community Mental Health Centers and the Treatment of Severe Mental Disorders," *American Journal of Psychiatry* 137 (1980): 83–86; Gerald N. Grob, *From Asylum to Community: Mental Health Policy in Modern America* (Princeton: Princeton University Press, 1991), 256–257.

9. Turner and TenHoor, "NIMH Community Support Program," 329, where the authors reference the National Institute of Mental Health–Community Support Section, *Request for Proposals*, NIMH no. MH-77-0080-0081, Rockville, Md., 1977), app. A, 1.

10. Richard C. Tessler and Howard H. Goldman, *The Chronically Mentally Ill: Assessing Community Support Programs* (Cambridge, Mass.: Ballinger, 1982), 12–13.

11. Turner and TenHoor, "NIMH Community Support Program," 326–327.

12. Ibid., 328–331.

13. Ibid., 323.

14. Ibid. The authors reference the General Accounting Office, *Returning the Mentally Disabled to the Community*, 36.

15. Tessler and Goldman, *The Chronically Mentally Ill*, 3–4.

16. Ibid., 3–4.

17. Howard H. Goldman and Antoinette A. Gattozzi, "Murder in the Cathedral Revisited: President Reagan and the Mentally Disabled," *Hospital & Community Psychiatry* 39 (1988): 505–509; Howard H. Goldman and Antoinette A. Gattozzi, "Balance of Powers: Social Security and the Mentally Disabled," *Milbank Quarterly* 66 (1988): 531–551; Leonard S. Rubenstein, Antoinette A. Gattozzi, and Howard H. Goldman, "Protecting the Entitlements of the Mentally Disabled: The SSDI/SSI Legal Battles of the 1980s," *International Journal of Law and Psychiatry* 11(1988): 269–278.

18. Koyanagi and Goldman, "Quiet Success of the National Plan," 899–903; Koyanagi and Goldman, *Inching Forward*, 15–34.

19. Ronald W. Reagan, "To the Congress of the United States," in *Fiscal Year 1982 Budget Revisions* (Washington, D.C.: Office of Management and Budget, Executive Office of the President, March 1981).

20. *Fiscal Year 1982 Budget Revisions: Additional Details on Budget Savings* (Washington, D.C.: Office of Management and Budget, Executive Office of the President, April 1981), 147.
21. Goldman and Gattozzi, "Murder in the Cathedral Revisited," 507.
22. M. E. Lando, A. V. Farley, and M. A. Brown, "Recent Trends in the Social Security Disability Program," *Social Security Bulletin* 45 (1982): 3–14.
23. Goldman and Gattozzi, "Murder in the Cathedral Revisited," 508; 98-1 Congress, *Social Security Disability Insurance: Hearing before the Subcommittee on Social Security of the Committee on Ways and Means, House of Representatives . . . June 30, 1983* (Washington, D.C.: Government Printing Office, 1983).
24. Goldman and Gattozzi, "Murder in the Cathedral Revisited," 506–508.
25. Ibid., 506.
26. 97-2 Congress, *Impact of the Accelerated Review Process on Cessations and Denials in the Social Security Disability Insurance Program: A Report by the Chairman of the Select Committee on Aging . . . House of Representatives . . . 1982* (Washington, D.C.: Government Printing Office, 1982).
27. Goldman and Gattozzi, "Murder in the Cathedral Revisited," 506.
28. 98-1 Congress, *Social Security Reviews of the Mentally Disabled: Hearings before the Special Committee on Aging . . . Senate . . . April 7 and 8, 1983* (Washington, D.C.: Government Printing Office, 1983), 119.
29. Rubenstein, Gattozzi, and Goldman, "Protecting the Entitlements," 271–273.
30. The following paragraphs on the legal battles involving Social Security are all documented in detail in Rubenstein, Gattozzi, and Goldman, "Protecting the Entitlements," 269–278.
31. Ibid., 271.
32. Ibid., 272.
33. Ibid.
34. Ibid., 275.
35. Goldman and Gattozzi, "Balance of Powers," 537–538; 98-1 Congress, *Social Security Reviews of the Mentally Disabled . . . 1983*.
36. Robert Pear, "Reagan Aide Hails Shift on Disability: Mrs. Heckler Says New Benefit Rules Will End Hardship—Health Units Disagree," *New York Times,* June 7, 1983, 1.
37. Goldman and Gattozzi, "Balance of Powers," 545–546.
38. Much of the material in the following paragraphs is based on the personal experience of one of the authors (HHG), who represented the National Institute of Mental Health as an assistant director on various Social Security Administration and American Psychiatric Association workgroups between 1983 and 1985.
39. Some of the details of the policy change are documented in Howard H. Goldman and Betty Runck, "Social Security Administration Revises Mental Disability Rules," *Hospital & Community Psychiatry* 36 (1985): 939–942.
40. Department of Health and Human Services, "Federal Old Age, Survivors, and Disability Insurance: Listings of Impairments—Mental Disorders. Final Rule," *Federal Register* 50 (1985): 35038–35070.
41. Koyanagi and Goldman, *Inching Forward,* 19.
42. Specific analysis of the DHHS Steering Committee, *National Plan for the Chronically Mentally Ill,* can be found in Koyanagi and Goldman, "Quiet Success of the National Plan," 899–903, and Koyanagi and Goldman, *Inching Forward,* 8. The SSA

recommendations can be found in the DHHS Steering Committee, *National Plan for the Chronically Mentally Ill*, 3-95.

43. Harold A. Pincus et. al., "Determining Disability Due to Mental Impairments: APA's Evaluation of Social Security Administration Guidelines," *American Journal of Psychiatry* 148 (1991): 1037–1043.

44. DHHS Steering Committee, *National Plan for the Chronically Mentally Ill*, 3-91.

45. Koyanagi and Goldman, "Quiet Success of the National Plan," 900, and Koyanagi and Goldman, *Inching Forward*, 8. The balance of this section is drawn from the analysis reported in these papers.

46. Koyanagi and Goldman, "Quiet Success of the National Plan," 902–903; Koyanagi and Goldman, *Inching Forward*, 34–45; Carl A. Taube, Howard H. Goldman, David Salkever, "Medicaid Coverage for Mental Illness: Balancing Access and Costs," *Health Affairs* 9 (1990): 19–30.

47. Daniel.S. Levine and Dorothy R. Levine, *The Cost of Mental Illness 1971*, NIMH Report Series B, no. 7 (Rockville, Md: ADAMHA, 1975), table 1.

48. Koyanagi and Goldman, "Quiet Success of the National Plan," 903; Koyanagi and Goldman, *Inching Forward*, 13.

49. Gerald N. Grob, *The Mad among Us: A History of the Care of America's Mentally Ill* (New York: Free Press, 1994), 284.

50. Taube, Goldman, and Salkever, "Medicaid Coverage for Mental Illness," 6–8; Richard G. Frank, Howard H. Goldman, and Michael Hogan, "Medicaid and Mental Health: Be Careful What You Ask For," *Health Affairs* 22 (2003): 101–113.

51. Koyanagi and Goldman, *Inching Forward*, 35, 41.

52. Koyanagi and Goldman, "Quiet Success of the National Plan," 901–903; Koyanagi and Goldman, *Inching Forward*, 34–45.

53. DHHS Steering Committee, *National Plan for the Chronically Mentally Ill*, 3-87. The strategy for the financing recommendations is laid out explicitly as an "incremental approach" on 3-45 through 3-51, including exhibits, followed by the thirteen Medicaid recommendations.

54. Koyanagi and Goldman, "Quiet Success of the National Plan," 901–903.

55. Koyanagi and Goldman, *Inching Forward*, 34–45.

56. Koyanagi and Goldman, "Quiet Success of the National Plan," 902, and Koyanagi and Goldman, *Inching Forward*, 39. The remainder of this section is derived from the analysis in *Inching Forward*.

57. Koyanagi and Goldman, *Inching Forward*, 36–37.

58. Legislation introduced by Senator John H. Chafee (R-RI) in the 101st Congress (S384).

59. Institute of Medicine, *Improving the Quality of Care in Nursing Homes*, a report from the Committee on Nursing Home Regulation (Washington, D.C.: National Academy of Sciences, 1986).

60. Koyanagi and Goldman, "Quiet Success of the National Plan," 902; Koyanagi and Goldman, *Inching Forward*, 9.

61. Antoinette A. Gattozzi and Howard H. Goldman, "IMD Classification," National Institute of Mental Health, Rockville, Md., 1986, mimeo, 1–3.

62. Jerry L. Mashaw and Virginia P. Reno, eds., *The Environment of Disability Income Policy: Programs, People, History, and Context*, Disability Panel Interim Report (Washington, D.C.: National Academy of Social Insurance, 1996), 76–78.

63. Judith R. Lave and Howard H. Goldman, "Medicare Financing for Mental Health Care," *Health Affairs* 9 (1990): 19–30.

64. See Koyanagi and Goldman, *Inching Forward,* 45–46, for more details on the benefit design.

65. Richard G. Frank and Thomas G. McGuire, "Economics and Mental Health," 894–954, in *Handbook of Health Economics,* ed. A. J. Culyer and J. P. Newhouse (Amsterdam: Elsevier, 2000).

66. Ed Hustead et al., "Reductions in Coverage for Mental and Nervous Illness in the Federal Employees Health Benefits Program: 1980–1984," *American Journal of Psychiatry* 142 (1985): 181–186.

67. DHHS Steering Committee, *National Plan for the Chronically Mentally Ill.*

68. Stephen F. Jencks et al, "Chapter 1: The Problem," in *Bringing Excluded Psychiatric Facilities under the Medicare Prospective Payment System: A Review of Research Evidence and Policy Options,* Supplement to *Medical Care* 25 (1987): S1–S5.

69. Ibid., S1.

70. Jencks et al., *Bringing Excluded Psychiatric Facilities,* S1–S51, provides the material used for the report to the Congress from the Department of Health and Human Services.

71. Some of the material in this section derives from the personal experience of one of the authors (HHG). From 1983 to 1985 he served as an assistant Institute director at the National Institute of Mental Health and chaired the ADAMHA Workgroup on Psychiatric Facilities under the Medicare Prospective Payment System.

72. These many studies are reviewed in Jencks et al., *Bringing Excluded Psychiatric Facilities,* particularly in Constance Horgan and Stephen F. Jencks, "Chapter 3: Research on Psychiatric Classification and Payment Systems," S22–S36.

73. Some of the key studies reviewed in Horgan and Jencks, "Chapter 3: Research on Psychiatric Classification and Payment Systems," include Marc Freiman et al., *A Study of Patient Classification Systems for Prospective Rate-Setting for Medicare Patients in Gneral Hospital Psychiatric Units and Psychiatric Hospitals,* Final Report on NIMH Contract 278-84-0011. (Silver Spring, Md.: Macro Systems, 1985); Joseph P. English et al., "Diagnosis-Related Groups and General Hospital Psychiatry: The APA Study," *American Journal of Psychiatry* 143 (1986): 131–139; and Dale M. Schumacher et al., "Prospective Payment for Psychiatry—Feasibility and Impact," *New England Journal of Medicine* 315 (1986): 1331–1336. The material in the Freiman et al. report appeared in several subsequent papers, including Marc Freiman et al., ""Simulating Policy Options for Psychiatric Care under Medicare's PPS," *Archives of General Psychiatry* 45 (1988): 1032–1036.

74. Judith R. Lave, "Developing a Medicare Prospective Payment System for Inpatient Psychiatric Care," *Health Affairs* 22 (2003): 97–109; "Medicare Program: Prospective Payment System for Inpatient Psychiatric Facilities. Final Rule," *Federal Register* 69 (2004): 66921–67015.

75. Howard H. Goldman, Gene D. Cohen, and Miriam Davis, "Economic Grand Rounds: Change in Medicare Outpatient Coverage for Alzheimer's Disease and Related Disorders," *Hospital & Community Psychiatry* 36 (1985): 939–942. This paper references the task force report and describes the process. The rest of the observations in this section derive from personal experience of one of the authors. During 1984–1985, Howard H. Goldman served as a consultant on financing policy issues to the task force.

76. Koyanagi and Goldman, *Inching Forward,* 47.

77. Steven S. Sharfstein and Howard H. Goldman, "Financing the Medical Management of Mental Disorders," *American Journal of Psychiatry* 146 (1989): 345–349.

78. Koyanagi and Goldman, "Quiet Success of the National Plan," 903, and Koyanagi and Goldman, *Inching Forward,* 47, are the sources for the remainder of the section on Medicare.

79. Koyanagi and Goldman, *Inching Forward,* 7.

80. Koyanagi and Goldman, *Inching Forward,* 59–60. The persistence of the problem of fragmentation is reflected in the interim and final reports of the 2002–2003 President's New Freedom Commission on Mental Health, discussed in more detail in the next chapter. President's New Freedom Commission on Mental Health, *Interim Report to the President* (Rockville, Md.: DHHS, October 2002), and President's New Freedom Commission on Mental Health. *Achieving the Promise: Transforming Mental Health Care in America,* Final Report (Rockville, Md.: DHHS, July 2003).

Chapter 6 — Integration, Parity, and Transformation

1. There are various papers that speak to these issues, including David Mechanic and David Rochefort, "Deinstitutionalization: An Appraisal of Reform," *Annual Review of Sociology* 16 (1990): 301–327; Linda Aiken, Stephen Somers, and Miles Shore, "Private Foundations in Health Affairs: A Case Study of a National Initiative for the Chronically Mentally Ill," *American Psychologist* 41 (1986): 1290–1295.

2. Chris Koyanagi and Howard H. Goldman, *Inching Forward: A Report on Progress Made in Federal Mental Health Policy in the 1980's* (Alexandria, Va.: National Mental Health Association, 1991), 7–53.

3. Joseph P. Morrissey and Howard H. Goldman, "Cycles of Reform in the Care of the Chronically Mentally Ill," *Hospital & Community Psychiatry* 35 (1984): 785–793.

4. Howard H. Goldman and Joseph P. Morrissey, "The Alchemy of Mental Health Policy: Homelessness and the Fourth Cycle of Reform," *American Journal of Public Health* 75 (1985): 727–731.

5. Howard H. Goldman, "The Program on Chronic Mental Illness," in *To Improve Health and Health Care 2000: The Robert Wood Johnson Foundation Anthology* ed. Stephen L. Isaacs and James R. Knickman (San Francisco: Jossey-Bass, 1999), 115–133. This retrospective look at the Robert Wood Johnson Foundation Program on Chronic Mental Illness provides an overview of the context for the demonstration and other mental health demonstration programs that followed.

6. Steven S. Sharfstein, Anne M. Stoline, and Howard H. Goldman, "Psychiatric Care and Health Insurance Reform," *American Journal of Psychiatry* 150 (1993): 7–18; Richard G. Frank, Howard H. Goldman, and Thomas G. McGuire, "Will Parity in Coverage Result in Better Mental Health Care," *New England Journal of Medicine* 345 (2001): 1701–1704.

7. Frank, Goldman, and McGuire, "Parity in Coverage," 1701–1704.

8. DHHS, *Mental Health: A Report of the Surgeon General* (Rockville, Md.: U.S. Public Health Service, 1999).

9. Tipper Gore's interest and involvement are described in a number of sources, including Jane Tanner, "Mental Health Insurance," *CQ Researcher* 12 (2002): 265–288, and Tipper Gore, "Children and Mental Illness," *National Forum* 73 (1993): 16–17.

10. Chris Koyanagi and Howard H. Goldman, "The Quiet Success of the National Plan for the Chronically Mentally Ill," *Hospital & Community Psychiatry* 42 (1991): 899–905; Goldman and Morrissey, "The Alchemy of Mental Health Policy," 727–731.

11. Koyanagi and Goldman, *Inching Forward*, 7–53.

12. Goldman, "The Program on Chronic Mental Illness," 122. As noted above, this source reviews the context for the program in the systems integration strategy of the times.

13. Koyanagi and Goldman, *Inching Forward*, 56.

14. Aiken, Somers, and Shore, "Private Foundations in Health Affairs," 1290–1295.

15. Ibid.; Mechanic and Rochefort, "Deinstitutionalization," 301–327.

16. Goldman, "The Program on Chronic Mental Illness," 121–122. See this source for more detailed references to the work of these other demonstration programs of this period.

17. Miles Shore and Martin D. Cohen, "The Robert Wood Johnson Foundation Program on Chronic Mental Illness: An Overview," *Hospital & Community Psychiatry* 41 (1990): 1212–1216.

18. Howard H. Goldman, Joseph P. Morrissey, and M. Susan Ridgely, "Form and Function of Mental Health Authorities at RWJ Foundation Program Sites: Preliminary Observations," *Hospital & Community Psychiatry* 41 (1990): 1222–1230.

19. Shore and Cohen, "Overview;" 1212–1214; Goldman, Morrissey, and Ridgely, "Form and Function," 1222–1228.

20. Goldman, "The Program on Chronic Mental Illness,"126.

21. Howard H. Goldman et al., "Design for the National Evaluation of the Robert Wood Johnson Foundation Program on Chronic Mental Illness," *Hospital & Community Psychiatry* 41 (1990): 1217–1221. The following description of the process for developing the demonstration evaluation comes in part from personal experience of one of the authors (HHG), who directed the evaluation during this period. The role of Carl A. Taube, mentioned in this section and later, also derives from personal experience. A brief description of Taube's contribution can be found in the introduction to a paper published posthumously: Carl A. Taube, Howard H. Goldman, and David Salkever, "Medicaid Coverage for Mental Illness: Balancing Access and Costs," *Health Affairs* 9 (1990): 19–30.

22. Goldman, "The Program on Chronic Mental Illness," 125–126.

23. Joseph P. Morrissey et al., "Mental Health Authorities and Service Systems Change from the RWJ PCMI," *Milbank Quarterly* 72 (1992): 49–80.

24. Richard G. Frank and Martin Gaynor, "Fiscal Decentralization of Public Mental Health Care and the Robert Wood Johnson Foundation Program on Chronic Mental Illness," *Milbank Quarterly* 72 (1992): 81–104.

25. Howard H. Goldman et al., "Lessons from the Evaluation of the Robert Wood Johnson Foundation Program on Chronic Mental Illness," *Health Affairs* 11 (1992): 51–68; Howard H. Goldman, Joseph P. Morrissey, and M. Susan Ridgely, "Evaluating the Robert Wood Johnson Foundation Program on Chronic Mental Illness (RWJ PCMI)," *Milbank Quarterly* 72 (1992): 37–48.

26. Anthony F. Lehman et al., "Continuity of Care and Clinical and Client Outcomes in the Robert Wood Johnson Foundation Program on Chronic Mental Illness," *Milbank Quarterly* 72 (1992): 105–122; David L. Shern et al., "Client Outcomes II: Longitudinal Client Data from the Colorado Treatment Outcome Study," *Milbank Quarterly* 72 (1992): 123–149.

27. Richard C. Tessler and Gail Gamache, "Continuity of Care, Residence, and Family Burden in Ohio," *Milbank Quarterly* 72 (1992): 149–170.

28. Sandra J. Neman et al., "The Effects of Independent Living on Persons with Chronic Mental Illness: An Assessment of the Section 8 Certificate Program," *Milbank Quarterly* 72 (1992): 171–198.

29. Goldman et al., "Lessons from the Evaluation," 51–65; Goldman, Morrissey, and Ridgely, "Evaluating the RWJ PCMI," 44.

30. M. Susan Ridgely et al., "Case Management and Client Outcomes in the Robert Wood Johnson Foundation Program on Chronic Mental Illness," *Psychiatric Services* 47 (1996): 737–743.

31. Goldman, "The Program on Chronic Mental Illness," 127.

32. Leonard Bickman, "A Continuum of Care: More Is Not Always Better," *American Psychologist* 51 (1996): 689–701.

33. Goldman, "The Program on Chronic Mental Illness," 127–131.

34. Ibid., 128. One of the Stewart B. McKinney Act programs is described in Robert Orwin et al., "Alcohol and Drug Abuse Treatment of Homeless Persons: Results from the NIAAA Community Demonstration Program," *Journal of Health Care for the Poor and Underserved* 5 (1994): 326–352.

35. Federal Task Force on Homelessness and Mental Illness, *Outcasts on Main Street,* ADM 92-1904 (Washington, D.C.: Interagency Council on the Homeless, 1992), 1–91.

36. Frances Randolph et al., "Creating Integrated Service Systems for Homeless Persons with Mental Illness: The ACCESS Program," *Psychiatric Services* 48 (1997): 369–373.

37. Joseph P. Morrissey et al., "Can Communities Improve Service Systems Integration for Homeless Persons with Serious Mental Illness? Evidence from the ACCESS Program," *Psychiatric Services* 53 (2002): 949–957.

38. Robert Rosenheck et al., "Do Efforts to Improve Service Systems Integration Enhance Outcomes for Homeless Persons with Serious Mental Illness? Evidence from the ACCESS Program," *Psychiatric Services* 53 (2002): 958–966.

39. Howard H. Goldman et al., "Lessons from the Evaluation of the ACCESS Program," *Psychiatric Services* 53 (2002): 967–969.

40. Bickman, "More Is Not Always Better," 689–701.

41. See *Schizophrenia Bulletin* 21 (1995) for several articles from the initial publications of the Schizophrenia PORT, including Anthony F. Lehman et al., "Treatment Outcomes in Schizophrenia: Implications for Practice, Policy, and Research," *Schizophrenia Bulletin* 21 (1995): 669–675.

42. Anthony F. Lehman, Donald M. Steinwachs, and the co-investigators of the PORT Project, "At Issue: Translating Research into Practice: The Schizophrenia Patient Outcomes Research Team (PORT) Treatment Recommendations," *Schizophrenia Bulletin* 24 (1998): 1–10.

43. DHHS, *Mental Health: A Report of the Surgeon General*; President's New Freedom Commission on Mental Health, *Interim Report to the President* (Rockville, Md.: DHHS, October, 2002), and President's New Freedom Commission on Mental Health, *Achieving the Promise: Transforming Mental Health Care in America. Final Report* (Rockville, Md.: DHHS, 2003).

44. Robert E. Drake et al., "Implementing Evidence-Based Practices in Routine Mental Health Service Settings," *Psychiatric Services* 52 (2001): 179–182, describes the

demonstration program. In 2001 the journal *Psychiatric Services* launched a series of papers on evidence-based practices, which are published together in Robert E. Drake and Howard H. Goldman, eds., *Evidence-Based Practices in Mental Health Care.* (Arlington, Va.: American Psychiatric Association, 2003). Another compendium on evidence-based practices is Robert E. Drake, ed., *Evidence-Based Practices in Mental Health Care* (Philadelphia: W. B. Saunders, 2003).

45. David Mechanic, *Mental Health and Social Policy: The Emergence of Managed Care,* 4th ed. (Boston: Allyn and Bacon, 1999); Dominic Hodgkin, "The Impact of Private Utilization Management on Psychiatric Care: A Review of the Literature," *Journal of Mental Health Administration* 19 (1992): 143–157; Susan M. Essock and Howard H. Goldman, "States' Embrace of Managed Care," *Health Affairs* 14 (1995): 1556–1558.

46. Bernard Arons et al., "Mental Health and Substance Abuse Coverage under National Health Reform," *Health Affairs* 13 (1994): 192–205; Howard H. Goldman, Richard G. Frank, nd Thomas G. McGuire, "Mental Health Care," in *Critical Issues in U.S. Health Reform,* ed. Eli Ginzberg (Boulder, Colo.: Westview Press, 1994), 73–92. Much of the material that follows in this section is based on the personal experience of one of the authors. During this period, HHG served as a consultant to the health care reform process. His observations are based on his own experiences and conversations with colleagues who were also involved, particularly Bernard Arons and Richard G. Frank. They all worked with Carl A. Taube, whose contribution to developing the field of mental health economics is also noted in the editor's introduction to Taube, Goldman, and Salkever, "Medicaid Coverage for Mental Illness."

47. Supported by a grant from the John D. and Catherine T. MacArthur Foundation, *Health Affairs* published a special section of papers on mental health policy in 1990 and 1992. The sections included the following papers on mental health care financing: Taube, Goldman and Salkever, "Medicaid Coverage for Mental Illness"; Judith R. Lave and Howard H. Goldman, "Medicare Financing for Mental Health Care," *Health Affairs* 9 (1990): 19–30; Richard G. Frank and Thomas G. McGuire, "Mandating Employer Coverage of Mental Health Care," ibid., 31–42; Richard G. Frank, Howard H. Goldman, and Thomas G. McGuire; "A Model Mental Health Benefit," ibid., 11 (1992): 98–117.

48. Robert Coulam and Joseph Smith, *Evaluation of the CPA—Norfolk Demonstration,* U.S. Defense Department Contract MDA 907-87-C-0003 (Cambridge, Mass.: Abt Associates, 1990).

49. Frank, Goldman, and McGuire, "Parity in Coverage," 1701–1702.

50. Joseph P. Newhouse, Insurance Experiment Group, *Free for All? Lessons from the RAND Health Insurance Experiment* (Cambridge: Harvard University Press, 1993).

51. Richard G. Frank and Thomas G. McGuire, "Economics and Mental Health," in *Handbook of Health Economics,* ed. A. J. Culyer and J. P. Newhouse (Amsterdam: Elsevier, 2000).

52. Ed Hustead et al., "Reductions in Coverage for Mental and Nervous Illness in the Federal Employees Health Benefits Program: 1980–1984," *American Journal of Psychiatry* 142 (1985): 181–186.

53. Goldman, Frank, and McGuire; "Mental Health Care," 80–84. See also Richard G. Frank and Thomas G. Mcguire, "Estimating Costs of Mental Health and Substance Abuse Coverage," *Health Affairs* 14 (1995): 102–115; Richard G. Frank,

Chris Koyanagi, and Thomas G. McGuire, "The Politics and Economics of Mental Health Parity Laws," *Health Affairs* 16 (1997): 108–120; Richard G. Frank et al., *Estimating the Costs of Parity for Mental Health: Methods and Evidence,* results from a Robert Wood Johnson Foundation workshop, Washington, D.C. (Princeton: Robert Wood Johnson Foundation, 2001).

54. As noted above, the description of the health care reform process is based on the personal experience of one of the authors (HHG) and conversations with participants.

55. Goldman, Frank, and McGuire, "Mental Health Care," 84–88, as well as in Arons et al., "Mental Health and Substance Abuse Coverage under National Health Reform," 192–205, and derived from Frank, Goldman, and McGuire, "A Model Mental Health Benefit," 98–117.

56. Much of the material in this section also appears in Howard H. Goldman and Gerald N. Grob, "Defining Mental Illness in Mental Health Policy," *Health Affairs,* 25 (2006): 737–749. The data come from Kevin D. Hennessy and Howard H. Goldman, "Full Parity: Steps Toward Treatment Equity for Mental and Addictive Disorders," *Health Affairs* 20 (2001): 58–67, and Marcia C. Peck and Richard M. Scheffler, "An Analysis of the Definition of Mental Illness Used in State Parity Laws," *Psychiatric Services* 53 (2002): 1089–1095.

57. Hennessy and Goldman, "Full Parity," 60–62; Peck and Scheffler, "Definition of Mental Illness on State Parity Laws," 1089–1094.

58. Frank, Goldman, and McGuire, "Parity in Coverage," 1701–1704.

59. C. Stephen Redhead, "Mental Health Parity Legislation," memorandum. Congressional Research Service, March 15, 2005, CRS-1–CRS-8.

60. General Accounting Office, *Mental Health Parity Act: Despite New Federal Standards Mental Health Benefits Remain Limited* (Washington, D.C.: General Accounting Office, 2000).

61. President Kennedy's directive to the Civil Service Commission is noted in Hustead et al., "Reductions in Coverage," 181–182, which also served as the source for the changes in federal employees' mental health benefits described in the balance of the paragraph.

62. Personal communication from Thomas Borneman, former deputy director of the Center for Mental Health Services, Substance Abuse and Mental Health Services Administration, DHHS, and from Tipper Gore. During this period author HHG served as senior scientific editor of the mental health report of the Surgeon General.

63. Office of the Press Secretary, White House, Press Release, "Resignation of Dr. Joycelyn Elders," December 9, 1994.

64. Office of the Vice President, Press Release, "Remarks of the President, the First Lady, the Vice President, and Mrs. Gore at the White House Conference on Mental Health," June 7, 1999.

65. DHHS, *Mental Health: A Report of the Surgeon General*; Robert Pear, "Mental Disorders Common, U.S. Says; Many Not Treated; Cost and Fear of Stigma Deter People from Effective Help, Surgeon General Says," *New York Times,* December 12, 1999, 1, 26. The balance of this section is based in part on the personal experiences of author HHG.

66. Howard H. Goldman, "Commentary: Making Culture Count in Mental Health Reports from the Surgeon General," *Culture, Medicine and Psychiatry* 27 (2003): 387–389. This commentary describes the conflict and its resolution.

67. DHHS, *Mental Health: Culture, Race and Ethnicity—A Supplement to Mental Health: A Report of the Surgeon General* (Rockville, Md.: U.S. Public Health Service, 2001).

68. The next section is based on the personal experience of author HHG and conversations with key actors, including Julius Richmond, M.D., and Surgeon General David Satcher, M.D., and his staff.

69. The policy recommendations were stated as "courses of action" in DHHS, *Mental Health: A Report of the Surgeon General*, "Chapter 8: A Vision of the Future," 451–458.

70. Michael F. Hogan, "The President's New Freedom Commission: Recommendations to Transform Mental Health Care in America," *Psychiatric Services* 54 (2003): 1467–1474.

71. Executive Order 13263, "President's New Freedom Commission on Mental Health," *Federal Register* 67 (May 3, 2002), actually issued April 29, 2002, in Albuquerque, New Mexico. The document can be found following 98 in President's New Freedom Commission on Mental Health, *Achieving the Promise*.

72. President's New Freedom Commission on Mental Health, *Achieving the Promise*. The report and its implications are described further in Ben C. Druss and Howard H. Goldman, "Introduction to the Special Section on the President's New Freedom Commission Report," *Psychiatric Services* 54 (2003): 1465–1466, and in Hogan, "Recommendations to Transform Mental Health Care in America," 1467–1474.

73. Executive Order 13263.

74. President's New Freedom Commission on Mental Health, *Achieving the Promise*; Substance Abuse and Mental Health Services Administration, U.S. Department of Health and Human Services, *Transforming Mental Health in America. Federal Action Agenda: First Steps*. DHHS Pub. no. SMA-05-4060 (Rockville, Md.: DHHS, 2005).

75. Hogan, "Recommendations to Transform Mental Health Care in America," 1467–1474; Druss and Goldman, "Introduction," 1465–1466.

76. Personal communication with Michael F. Hogan, October 2002.

77. President's New Freedom Commission on Mental Health, *Interim Report.*

78. Personal communication, informal remarks made by Rosalynn Carter at a dinner meeting of the President's New Freedom Commission on Mental Health, February 4, 2003, Washington, D.C.

79. President's New Freedom Commission on Mental Health, *Achieving the Promise*, 1–86.

80. Responses from the key members of the Campaign for Mental Health are reported in *Psychiatric Services* 54 (2003): Robert W. Glover, "Statement from the National Association of State Mental Health Program Directors," ibid., 1477; Robert Bernstein, "Statement from the Bazelon Center for Mental Health Law," ibid., 1477–1478; Michael Faenza, "Statement from the National Mental Health Association," ibid., 1478–1479; Richard Birkel, "Statement from the National Alliance for the Mentally Ill," ibid., 1479.

81. Howard H. Goldman et al., "Behavioral Health Insurance Parity for Federal Employees," *New England Journal of Medicine* 354, no. 13 (March 30, 2006): 1378–1386.

82. DHHS, *Transforming Mental Health in America*, Preface.

83. Campaign for Mental Health Reform, *Emergency Response: A Roadmap for Federal Action in America's Mental Health Crisis* (Washington, D.C.: The Campaign, July 2005). See also www.info@mhreform.org.

Epilogue

1. Richard G. Frank and Sherry A. Glied, *Better but Not Well* (Baltimore, Md.: Johns Hopkins University Press, 2006).

2. Executive Order 13263, "President's New Freedom Commission on Mental Health," *Federal Register* 67 (May 3, 2002), actually issued April 29, 2002, in Albuquerque, New Mexico. The document can be found following 98 in President's New Freedom Commission on Mental Health, *Achieving the Promise.* The question is from sec. 3, "Mission."

Index

Aarons, Bernard, 161, 165, 213n46

ACCESS. *See* Access to Community Care and Effective Services and Supports

Access to Community Care and Effective Services and Supports, evaluation, 158–159, 160

Achieving the Promise: Transforming Mental Health Care in America (2003), 160, 177, 184

ACT. *See* Assertive Community Treatment

Action for Mental Health (1961), 28, 32, 37

Ad Hoc Committee on the Chronic Mental Patient, 81

ADAMHA. *See* Alcohol, Drug Abuse, and Mental Health Administration

AFDC. *See* Aid to Families with Dependent Children

African Americans, 93

AFSCME. *See* American Federation of State, County, and Municipal Employees

aged, 48–49, 88, 95; in mental hospitals, 8–9

Agency for Health Care Policy and Research, 159, 161

AHCPR. *See* Agency for Health Care Policy and Research

AHRQ. *See* Agency for Healthcare Research and Quality

Aid to Families with Dependent Children, 133, 135, 139

Aiken, Linda, 152

Alaskan Natives, 93

Albee, George W., 54, 81–82, 87

Alcohol, Drug Abuse, and Mental Health Administration, 140, 157; and Mental Health Services Block Grant, 151

Allan, Priscilla, 72, 77, 81, 86–87, 91–92

Alliance for the Liberation of Mental Patients, 79

almshouses, persons with mental illnesses in, 8

Alzheimer's disease, 138, 143–145

Ambrose, John, 107

American Federation of State, County, and Municipal Employees, 107, 111

American Hospital Association, 26, 107, 141

American Medical Association, 26, 41; reaction to *Action for Mental Health,* 31; opposes staffing subsidies for CMHCs, 38

American Nurses'Association, 107

American Occupational Therapy Association, 107

American Psychiatric Association, 14, 26, 106, 141; and reorientation of post World War II psychiatry, 16; Central Inspection Board, 17; Mental Hospital Institutes, 17; reaction to *Action for Mental Health,* 30–31; report on homeless persons with mental disorders, 58; and President's Commission on Mental Health, 74, 82, 98–99; conference on chronic patients, 81; and patient bill of rights, 110–111; and disability reviews, 128

American Psychological Association, 106; reaction to *Action for Mental Health,* 31

anti-psychiatry movement, 53–56

Appel, Kenneth E., 26

Appelbaum, Paul S., 56

Asia/Pacific Island Americans, 88, 93

Assertive Community Treatment, 153, 159

Association for the Advancement of Psychology, 106

Bazalon Center for Mental Health Law, 128, 178

Bedlam 1946 (Maisel), 16–17

Beigel, Alan, 72, 81, 91

bill of rights, patient, 110–112

Birnbaum, Morton, 54

birth rate, rise in, 57

Black Americans, 88

Bond, Kit, 175

Boston Psychopathic Hospital, 22, 48

Bourne, Peter, 69

Gerald N. Grob is the Henry E. Sigerist Professor of the History of Medicine Emeritus at Rutgers University in New Brunswick, N.J. His specialty is the history of mental health policy. He has written more than fifty articles and has authored or edited more than a dozen volumes. His major work is a three-volume history of mental health policy (*Mental Institutions in America: Social Policy to 1875* [1973], *Mental Illness and American Society 1875–1940* [1983], and *From Asylum to Community: Mental Health Policy in Modern America* [1991]). His one volume comprehensive history, *The Mad Among Us: A History of the Care of America's Mentally Ill* was published in 1994. He is an elected member of the Institute of Medicine of the National Academy of Sciences, and has held Guggenheim and other fellowships as well as NIMH research grants. His most recent book is *The Deadly Truth: A History of Disease in America* (2002).

Howard H. Goldman, M.D., Ph.D., is professor of psychiatry at the University of Maryland School of Medicine in Baltimore, MD. His specialty is mental health policy research. He has written more than two hundred and fifty articles and has authored or edited ten volumes. He was the Senior Scientific Editor of *Mental Health: A Report of the Surgeon General* (1999) and a consultant to the President's New Freedom Commission on Mental Health (2002–2003). He is an elected member of the Institute of Medicine of the National Academy of Sciences and an elected member of the National Academy of Social Insurance. Dr. Goldman is editor-in-chief of Psychiatric Services, a journal of mental health services and policy research published by the American Psychiatric Association.